Roots and New Frontiers in Social Group Work

About the Editors

Marcos Leiderman, MSW, MCRP, is Professor of group work at Rutgers University School of Social Work at New Brunswick, New Jersey. As a member of the Board of State Health Council, he has been making policy decisions on health care for the region for nine years. Professor Leiderman has published articles in the areas of mental health, social work, and health planning.

Martin Birnbaum, PhD, is an academician and group work consultant. As an adjunct professor at Rutgers University Graduate School of Social Work, he teaches group work theory and practice. He provides in-service training and group supervision to group work agencies and enables case work oriented agencies to develop and institutionalize group work services.

Barbara Dazzo, MSW, PhD, is a member of the adjunct faculty of both the Rutgers School of Social Work and the Robert Wood Johnson Medical School. She has extensive experience in individual, group, and family modalities, and in conducting group training workshops here and abroad. She has published in the areas of social services and human sexuality.

Roots and New Frontiers in Social Group Work

*Selected Proceedings
Seventh Annual Symposium on the
Advancement of Social Work with Groups*

Edited by
Marcos Leiderman
Martin L. Birnbaum
Barbara Dazzo

The Haworth Press
New York • London

Roots and New Frontiers in Social Group Work is supplement #3 to *Social Work with Groups*. It is not supplied as part of the subscription to the journal, but is available from the publisher at an additional charge.

The Haworth Press, Inc., 12 West 32 Street, New York, NY 10001
EUROSPAN/Haworth, 3 Henrietta Street, London WC2E 8LU England

LIBRARY OF CONGRESS
Library of Congress Cataloging-in-Publication Data

Symposium on the Advancement of Social Work with Groups (7th : 1985 :
  Rutgers University)
    Roots and new frontiers in social group work : selected proceedings / Seventh Annual Symposium on the Advancement of Social Work with Groups; edited by Marcos Leiderman, Martin L. Birnbaum, Barbara Dazzo.
       p. cm. — (Supplement #3 to Social work with groups, ISSN 0897-8441)
    Includes bibliographies.
    ISBN 0-86656-727-5
    1. Social group work — Congresses. 2. Social group work — United States — Congresses. I. Leiderman, Marcos. II. Birnbaum, Martin L. III. Dazzo, Barbara. IV. Title. V. Series: Supplement . . . to Social work with groups : #3.
HV45.S95   1985
361.4 — dc19   88-529
                                                                                      CIP

Selected Proceedings
Seventh Annual Symposium on the
Advancement of Social Work with Groups

EXECUTIVE BOARD
OF THE COMMITTEE FOR THE ADVANCEMENT
OF SOCIAL WORK WITH GROUPS

SYMPOSIUM ORGANIZING COMMITTEE

SYMPOSIUM PROGRAM COMMITTEE

Barbara Dazzo, Chairperson

Martin L. Birnbaum,
Abstract Selection Committee

David Blevins,
Finance and Budget Committee

Leonard Brown,
Audio Visual Committee

Leslie Friedman,
Exhibitions Committee

Len Kates,
Evaluation Committee

Maria Katonak,
Special Events Committee

Larry Lamson
Historical Exhibit Committee

Sr. Julie Scanlan, S. C.
Testimonials and Honors
Committee

Wilma Selenfriend,
Institute Committee

David Stern,
Fund Raising Committee

Constance Stober,
Registration Committee

Irene Stolzenberg,
Hospitality Committee

William L. Tatum, Jr.,
Symposium Coordinator

Ceil Miller
Executive Assistant to
Symposium Chairperson

HONOREES

Dorothy Height
Celine Marcus
Rose Movitch
Marjorie Murphy
Julius Samuels
Sanford Solender

TESTIMONIALS

Terence Cardinal Cooke
Clara Kaiser
Arnulf Pins
Gertrude Wilson

CONTENTS

THEORY AND RESEARCH

ISSUES AND TRENDS IN GROUP WORK THEORY,
PRACTICE AND EDUCATION

Foreword

These selected Proceedings bring to us only a brief glimpse of the richness and expansiveness of the 7th Annual Symposium on the Advancement of Social Work with Groups, held at Rutgers University in 1985. Through the splendid efforts of the Organizing and Program Committees under the leadership of the Chairperson, Marcos Leiderman, Symposium VII captured with new vigor the heritage of social group work. Sometimes this has seemed lost as practice becomes more complex and social group work education seeks to provide enlightenment for the present and future. We are indebted to the planners of this Symposium for bringing us closer to understanding the relationship of our origins to more recent developments and potentials.

Social Work with Groups will continue to participate in the renaissance of group work in our profession as it is reflected in the Annual Symposia and the published proceedings. This publication enhances the tradition.

Catherine Papell

Preface

The year 1985 witnessed the 7th Consecutive Symposium of the Committee for the Advancement of Social Work with Groups (CASWG), sponsored by Rutgers University School of Social Work, New Brunswick, New Jersey.

The Symposium was organized and conducted for professional social workers working with Groups from across the United States, Canada, England and other European Countries including Israel.

The theme of the 7th Symposium — Roots and New Frontiers — celebrated the first one hundred years of social group work, marked by the 100th anniversary of Toynbee Hall in London and University Settlement in the United States. The Symposium focused on a continuum of social group work from its historical beginnings to present day practice and toward an innovative view of future practice. It links the origin of social group work to its present and future frontiers.

For several decades, practitioners in settlement, Y's and community centers, recreation, camping and adult education programs practiced group work, and developed and integrated a theoretical foundation for diverse practice concepts. Margaret Berry, in a recent publication on the one hundred years of urban frontiers documents the beginnings of group work in the settlement movement, 1886-1986. She states, "Of all the specializations, the strongest affinity was with social group work because of its relevance to settlement values — its emphasis on human relationships and on democratic decision making including social action."[1]

From the settlements, social group work derived its institutional

---

[1]Margaret E. Berry, "One Hundred Years of Urban Frontiers: The Settlement Movement, 1886-1986," published for the 1986 Centennial of the U.S. Settlement Movement by United Neighborhood Centers of America, 1319 F., N.W. 10, Suite 603, Washington, D.C. 20004.

base. Its leadership was committed to the development of responsible citizenship, acculturation, participation in the democratic process and collective action and a solidarity that helped translate the nation's promise for freedom, opportunity and dignity into reality for its diverse populations.

The New Frontiers Theme is a link to the newer trends in social work with groups. The symposium covered a wide range and diversity of group work, practice, theory, research and education. Papers and presentations included content on health and mental health institutions, substance abuse programs, rehabilitation centers, the correctional system, family service agencies, nursing homes. Newer specialized areas included fields like industry, victims of child and spouse abuse, and incest.

Some of the outstanding features of this symposium were: (1) It was a grass roots undertaking planned in three regions, New Jersey, New York and Pennsylvania, engaging educators and practitioners not usually involved in the symposiums; (2) It attracted a large number of social group workers from foreign countries who shared the similarities and differences of their experiences. (3) The Board of CASWG in collaboration with those attending the symposium amended the bylaws converting the committee to a membership organization; and (4) A major historical exhibit celebrated the first hundred years of Toynbee Hall, a settlement house in London, England and the University Settlement in New York City.

We wish to thank all of the planning committee members, and all of those who contributed to the success of the symposium. We extend special thanks to Dean Harold Demone, Rutgers University, School of Social Work and the faculty and staff for their support; Virginia Lee Lusier, Assistant Provost; Joe Czapp, Director of Continuing Education; and Ceil Miller, Executive Secretary. We wish to recognize the editorial contributions of Sr. Julie Scanlan, S.C., and extend our grateful appreciation to her.

Marcos Leiderman
Chairperson, Editorial Committee

Introduction

The Selected Papers reflect the themes of the Symposium: Roots and New Frontiers. Wohl, the keynote speaker, tracing the roots of the settlement movement and group work discusses the plight of the modern human being in the struggles of their urban environment. He presents a framework for looking at society through the analysis of our past and present strategies of social group work intervention. Wohl stresses the widespread neglect of social responsibility, social action and social change. He suggests that in order to solve social problems, it is necessary to choose crucial factors, to partialize the issues and to become active problem solvers in the front line of the battle against poverty, racism, sexism and ageism. He stresses that social workers with groups in liaison with other fighters carry frontier responsibilities in our communities. The speaker provides excerpts from his own practice in a neighborhood settlement house in the West side of Manhattan, illustrating the practical application of his theoretical beliefs.

The articles in the section on group work practice deal with group work services for populations that don't easily fit into services provided by the community — the deinstitutionalized, homeless; mentally ill adults in aftercare; families who care for schizophrenic members; troubled children and teenagers who need therapeutic services during the summer. The programs are reminiscent of our roots and beginnings in settlement houses, recreation, and education. They serve the client's needs for socialization, empowerment, education and support. James Forte's paper on a new age settlement house is a remarkable demonstration of group work programming that fosters individual well-being while at the same time motivates the homeless and downtrodden to engage in social action to change the community in which they live through self-help and mutual aid groups. Margaret Lazar's families of chronically ill adults are empowered through education and support groups. The integration of activities into treatment approaches for populations that are less able to benefit from verbal interactions and reflection are described and discussed for two divergent populations. Hitchcock deals with group treatment that fosters social skills, problem solving and independence in chronically mentally ill adults while Weiland, Zafran and Brooks discuss group work in a therapeutic summer camp for clients from a community mental health center. The names of the populations have changed, but the unique perspective of social group work as a method that enhances independence and autonomy in the individual, through participation in a mutual aid process, remains the same. The use of natural helping networks as a therapeutic milieu for problem employees seems to be a natural extension of social group work into industrial settings. Aschner's groups in industry explores the growth and development of this new frontier and the effective use of groups in this setting. The final paper in this section, Annie Wu King's piece on Chinese painting, is a practitioner's look at how her own "ethnicity" influences her approach to treatment, and how this suggests the possibility of growth for ourselves as professionals.

The collection of articles in the education and training section deals with issues both in the classroom and in the field of practice. Gladstein has written an insightful analysis on how the group is used to help students when crisis arises in their field placements. Using examples of a work stoppage and strike, the students are exposed to a mutual aid group which helps them to process conflictual values and ethical issues resulting from unionization of professional social workers.

Levin's paper reflects the process of change in participants attending a workshop dealing with the nuclear threat. The model for the "changing the silence" workshop is "despair and empowerment." The group experience demonstrates on how the numbing of fear and helplessness can be transformed into personal power and social change. It is their first opportunity to speak about living with the nuclear threat. The article, "Teaching Group Work Skills Through Reflection-in-Action," by Getzel addresses the question of how faculty and students can use the record of service as an instrument to collaboratively examine their mutual understanding of the ongoing practice issues. Getzel describes different types of records of service and explores how students can use them to identify specific problems. He also presents the concept of reflection-in-action that can be used to think about practice. Weil's paper, "Task Group Skills: The Core of Community Practice," points out the need for a renewed understanding of the task group in community organization. Weil calls for a refocusing on the common grounding of values, process and skills for community practice which need to be stressed in the education of students and in the training of practitioners.

The current trend to provide training at the workplace for professionals, is reflected in Brown's paper, "Staff Groups: Creative Problem Solving in the Workplace" where he uses the group as a framework for growth and change. Brown contributes a model for reducing stress and for enhancing wellness for social workers and other human service personnel in a hospital setting through the development of staff groups. He helps to identify the major stressors on the job and he offers practical ways in which the group can be used for problem solving and stress reduction.

The section on theory and research offers two different studies on the state of the art in social work with groups. The opening article, by Goldberg and Lamont, focuses on the effects of the shift from a method specialization curriculum to an integrated one and the effect this shift had on the students' knowledge and skill levels in social group work at Wayne State University. The impact of the loss of the old sequence structure has had its greatest effect on the student's inability in maintaining familiarity with the group work literature. The findings point in two opposite directions. While the subjects perceive that their skills of competency with groups has declined the interest and practice opportunities in the field persists. The paper by Singer et al. is a fine example of action research. The authors show how a demonstration research project is used to enhance the social environment in an institution for the elderly. The power of the small group for support, problem solving and social action is demonstrated as residents, staff and families interact around their common needs and concerns. The final paper in this section by Seebaldt deals with the value conflicts of the professional helper. It provides a conceptual framework for self-awareness. The personal values regarding the problem and the reality of their authority in the group, is explored as a primary factor in helping group decision making. It also enables the group members to bring forth their operative values and help them make choices from alternatives that are fully human rather than just expedient.

The final section of the selected papers, issues and trends in group work theory, education and practice address some common concerns affecting the future development of social group work. The authors are concerned with the curriculum changes in schools of social work that have eliminated group work as a major in most graduate schools that have relegated group work courses to electives and de-emphasized group work content within generic courses. They address the serious implications of these changes for social work education and practice and call for putting group work content back into the social work curriculum. Another common concern centers on the issue of how group work is currently practiced. They stress the importance of social work with groups as embracing group process as the power in producing change in the individual and empowering the group. They indicate an optimism about the resurgence of social group work through the development of the *Journal of Social Work with Groups*, The Committee for the Advancement of Social Work with Groups, and the Annual Group Work Symposia.

Goldberg's paper, "Breaking the Thought Barriers: New Frontiers in Social Work with Groups," challenges us to change our modes of thinking and to become aware of the barriers to expanded thinking about social work with groups. For example, in order to reverse the trends in social work education we need to destroy the idea that the generic/generalist orientation to teaching social work is sufficient preparation for group work practice.

Lewis describes the findings of a curriculum study she conducted on education for social group work practice. The data supports the contention that social work practice with groups is a neglected entity in the curriculum. She makes a compelling case for adding theory and practice with groups to all of social work education showing how prevention, empowerment, problem solving and support are enhanced through group activity.

In their paper, Middleman and Goldberg explore the criteria for social work practice with groups in order to distinguish social group work from other forms of group practice. The authors examine current trends in relation to open-ended groups, single session groups and self-help groups and also identify issues and directions for research.

Martin L. Birnbaum
Barbara Dazzo
Marcos Leiderman

Keynote Address

Roots and New Frontiers

Bernard J. Wohl

SUMMARY. A keynote speech of the 7th Annual Symposium on the Advancement of Social Work with Groups discusses the contemporary social political climate of 1985 in which there has been a retreat to privatism by social workers and other professionals. By examining the development of social group work through its roots with emphasis on social concerns and social action the author rekindles a torch illuminating the human condition in our society. He stresses the responsibility of social workers with groups in becoming active problem solvers of issues compounded by poverty, racism and sexism.

We are meeting at a time of throwback, of the systematic destruction of the concept of social welfare. The administration under which we live pursues a policy of bold regression to destroy historic achievements. It is difficult and fearsome to oppose the ethos projected by one's ruling government. It is easier to retreat to privatism.

Bernard J. Wohl, Executive Director, Goodard-Riverside Community Center, New York, N.Y.

This is not a problem faced by social workers alone. For every calling that has a passion of purpose, there is a crisis today. In an address to young writers last spring, E. L. Doctorow said: "ironically in our withdrawal, our non-political, pragmatic vision of ourselves and our calling, we may be expressing the general crisis of our age, we are writing as we live, in a kind of stunned submission to the political circumstances of our lives and the establishmentarian rule of our politicians. We are being bought off by our comfort while great moral outrages are committed in our name." He reaches back to the masters of writing for other patterns.

The history of the settlement house movement and its passionate group workers has something to say to us today about strength and tenacity in the struggle for social welfare.

In this address, I will be weaving back and forth between our historic roots and the new challenges we face.

Many of the root issues addressed by the historic settlement houses – Toynbee Hall, Hull House, University Settlement, The College Settlements, Andover House, Henry Street – are still with us but have undergone the smashing sea change of history. Poverty and discrimination, the bestialities against children, the garbage in the poorer wards, the humiliation of women and the fight for women's suffrage, the struggle to organize an international crusade for peace and the defeat of that struggle in the outbreak of World War I and the war's aftermath of a poisoned peace stretched every sinew of the early social workers. They won some battles and they lost more but they left a heritage – some victories in legislation and social structures, some local successes – Jane Addams got to be the Inspector of Garbage Removal in her ward – as well as much later and perhaps most important a commitment to values that nourished a philosophy of human life and created a vision.

The early social workers worked with every kind of group – small groups for sewing, for reading the classics, for learning English and citizenship, for local community improvement in housing and health. They worked in liaison with other groups and organizations, unions and churches and colleges. They also left a heritage of courage and integrity in defeat as well as in victory.

Early American settlement leaders, Stanton Coit, Robert A. Woods, Charles Stover, Jane Addams, Mary Simkovitch, and others were deeply affected by the poverty they witnessed in the London slums as well as in their own neighborhoods, and viewed the Toynbee Hall settlement idea as a step in reforming the social malaise of the city dwellers.

Most of the pioneer initiators of the American settlement movement were women. The College Settlements Association, which was to sponsor five houses in rapid succession, was inaugurated by a small group of Smith College Alumnae in 1887. In 1888 Jane Addams and Ellen Starr visited Toynbee Hall and in so doing crystallized their determination to rent a house in a part of Chicago where needs cried out for resources and solutions. Both College Settlement on Rivington Street in New York City and Hull House in Chicago were started in 1889. Andover House in Boston was founded in 1891. Additional College Settlements were founded in Philadelphia in 1892, Henry Street in New York in 1893, and College Settlement in Los Angeles in 1894. The significant fact about the establishment of this group of nine pioneer houses is that they were initiated, sponsored, governed, staffed and supported by women. Jane Addams went to some pains to make clear why this was so. She defined the urge to social action as desire "to share the life of the human race." She wrote that "settlement workers are bound to regard the entire life of their city as organic, to make an effort to unify it, and to protect against its over differentiation." This over differentiation included the sphere of action of women, and in a paragraph classifying the activities of Hull House as social, educational, humanitarian and civic, she adds the qualifying rider, "if indeed a settlement of women can be said to have civic responsibilities."

Her account of an incident at the first White House Conference on Children in 1909 links the two great minorities of the period. A young military aide of the President had been put in charge of five speakers for the mass meeting at which Theodore Roosevelt was to preside with instructions that the panel was to file upon the platform at the exact moment the President started down the main aisle. The young man was nervous lest his charges get out of order, and as the zero moment approached, he was overheard to mutter, counting them off on his fingers, "I have my Protestant, my Catholic, my Jew, my Negro and the woman." Booker T. Washington facing around said, "I am very sorry to take precedence over you, Miss Addams, but I can assure you it is the first time in my life that I have not been at the end of the line." Jane Addams replied, "Make no mistake Mr. Washington, the woman is always last." The women's settlements lifted the feminist movement out of a doctrinaire campaign into the beginnings of a social force. Hull House was perhaps the foremost feminist enclave in the world. The women Miss Addams gathered about her included Grace and Edith Abbott, Alice Hamilton and Frances Perkins who became leaders of the legislative and social reform movement for the next 40 years. The suffragist movement and the role of women during war time emanated from the settlement house movement.

The philosophy of the settlement movement led to reform as well as philanthropy. The settlement residents were early "lobbyists" who fought hard for federal and state protective legislation. They influenced passage of child labor laws, a minimum wage bill, and better conditions and shorter hours for women. They were also instrumental in the labor union movement and assisted in its early struggles. They realized that not to get involved in the struggle to improve economic conditions would be remiss. Settlements served as meeting places for the labor unions. With the ushering in of the Progressive Era in the United States, settlements sharpened their focus on the national level. Although their leaders had already helped organize such national organizations as the National Child Labor Committee, the National Women's Trade Union League and the NAACP, settlement workers yearned for other organized expressions of social reform as well. They threw their weight behind Theodore Roosevelt and the Progressive Party in 1912 with its planks of social and industrial reform.

In the years before World War I, Jane Addams and her associates were deeply committed to the international struggles for peace and disarmament. When those struggles were lost, she continued to oppose the war and the repression which followed. But in this she was among the loners. Many other social workers accommodated the war and its aftermath. The major thrust of the United States settlements began to change. Many felt that their primary responsibility was "to provide major leisure activities and to teach art and dramatics to all who were interested." Settlements like the rest of America, were lulled into a sense of security and prosperity. Nevertheless, the problems of slum living and the need to service poor immigrants remained, even during the national prosperity of the post-war world. By the time the depression of the 1930s developed, many of the settlement houses, under the leadership of the National Federation of Settlements (now United Neighborhood Centers of America formed in 1911), became actively involved, first in the pre-Roosevelt efforts and then in the New Deal. Some settlement members sat on the advisory council of the President's Committee on Economic Security which led to the formulation of the Social Security Act of 1935.

The 40s and 50s saw the advent of the psychoanalytic school of psychology and its influence on social group work. The therapeutic model was the modality of the decade. To be sure there were group work agencies that were deeply involved politically in struggling for public housing, in voicing their concern about the growing drug abuse malady among teens, in accelerated school attrition, in developing preschool programs for working mothers — however, the focus of most group work agencies was on recreation for the youth and adults of poorer communities.

The 60s and 70s in group work literature were "characterized by the development and refinement of differing conceptual models of practice . . . it was clear that [group work] had dropped the emphasis on education and had become identified with social work with a concomitant emphasis on treatment and rehabilitation. Democratic participation and social change remained somewhat in the background. . . ." And yet our world was changing.

Problems of change are problems of choice and inherent in making the choice, particularly in those years, was conflict. As the developing nations emerged from colonialism, consciousness of change was also felt in the "dependent" areas of the United States. The black people of Birmingham, Alabama, knew the world was changing and wanted their world changed too. And they attempted to change it. There were those who were profoundly disturbed at witnessing thousands of blacks in the United States out on the streets in an open struggle against segregation and indignity; on one side of the conflict — white police, dogs, and monitored hoses which could strip bark off trees at a hundred feet; on the other side, blacks joined in the early days of the civil rights struggle by white activists who rejected racism. The critics of the conflict wanted to mute it, to slow the pace. They wanted the blacks to go slower, to do it differently, to be quieter, to choose another method, to inch forward for another hundred years. But in a world in which ten year time tables put astronauts on the moon, human rights in the millennium were unappealing. That was the field of discrimination.

Now let's take hunger. All say hunger is evil and that human beings must eat. But there are differences as to how soon, how much, and out of whose trough. Hunger still rides a pale horse in parts of the United States. Michael Harrington's book, *The Other America* and the War on Poverty had a profound effect on the settlements. They were forced to take their place among a barrage of agencies. Massive government funding of other forms of community programs mitigated the unique role of the settlement house. By 1967 there were 1600 neighborhood centers and 700 neighborhood legal offices outside the settlement house establishment. Mobilization for Youth, precursor of the community action agency, ironically owed its beginnings to Henry Street Settlement and the efforts of Helen Hall. Then MFY became a critic of the settlements. It viewed them as "being essentially antiquated and irrelevant." Community action agencies considered the settlements establishment-oriented, conservative forces in the neighborhood. Most of the settlements throughout the country contracted for specific services and did not get involved in social action programs.

Let me attempt to develop my own analysis of where we are going based on this history. Today's settlement workers—those who are the closest to the slum dweller and the poor of the cities have seen the poor primarily as individuals and individual families but not in their social presence—in their common problem and common power. We talk of community organization but we seldom mean by that organizing the unemployed, the mother on welfare, the disadvantaged minorities. Social action is all too often restricted to well-controlled committee meetings and the adroit contributions of a central lobbyist.

Today's settlement workers understand, will speak for and write about the need for adequate welfare standards, minority rights, jobs for youth, but they seldom see as part of their job helping to orga-

nize the unorganized low-income and welfare families in their settlement areas, helping them to articulate their hurts, define their
needs and express their desires, help them find their own forms of
organization and constructive leadership, and help them to use the
only resource they have, themselves, their sheer existence, their
love of life, their desire to live and achieve their aspirations. This is
a major asset of the poor and the minority person. We have not
tapped it.

The settlement worker in today's setting of change has not played
a role in organizing the unorganized because we have not yet decided what we ought to be doing about this in our place in the urban
whirlpool.

The Reagan administration exacerbates our problems. It is now
clear that the multi-billion dollar Reagan budget deficits were created deliberately to cut the social programs and services his administration intended to cut. It is much easier for the administration to
argue that we cannot afford basic programs than to argue that the
programs themselves are not worthwhile.

The President blames the deficit crisis on excessive domestic
spending despite the fact that from 1982 to 1985 he has reduced
domestic spending drastically and escalated defense spending.

The tax giveaways combined with massive increases in military
expenditures created the deficit crisis. One of the basic post-elec-
tion issues is the role of the middle class and the poor in defending
Social Security, Medicare, Medicaid and food stamps. Where are
the settlements and other group serving agencies in this situation?
What are we doing in our cities throughout the nation? With whom
are we aligning ourselves? Let me return for a minute to history.

Jane Addams reported a peace conference — one she helped organize — where the question was raised: why do those who advocate
the conscription of life oppose the socialization of wealth? And
might not future wars be prevented if property was conscripted simultaneously with young men? Hull House in its day sheltered un-
popular causes and suffered adverse criticism. It was not Hull
House alone. Lillian Wald in *Windows on Henry Street* wrote of her
work for peace during World War I and reported how she was "dis-
ciplined by the torture chamber method of having the money with-

drawn which enabled the nurses to care for the families of the soldiers no less than the other sick.''

Helen Hall in 1936 also dealt with these sensitive and eruptive problems in her article, ''The Consequences of Social Action for the Group Work Agency.'' Writing of the need to turn ''our social concern into social action,'' she declared: ''. . . it is poor group work to leave the groups one deals with unconscious of the part they can play in changing their own living conditions. Groups of tenement mothers organized by settlements in New York have for years been going to Albany to testify as to tenement conditions. As consumers of housing they bring a reality and detail that none of the rest of us can match . . .''

''There are two kinds of consequences involved in social action,'' Helen Hall explains, ''first, the gains or setbacks to the community; second, the consequences to the social agency itself . . .''

''As social workers we can bear in mind that one of the telling forces in securing the enactment of relief and social security legislation was the demand of the unemployed themselves. Their processions, their meetings, their delegations to Washington — all counted in the momentum that dislodged our national inertia. Social action for change is inescapable unless we are willing to drift along eternally patching up the consequences of social neglect and industrial breakdown. We should share in it and help shape it, but increasingly the force that is going to count most will be made up of the people most concerned, and as group working agencies we can help keep the channels open for education and expression so that there is better equipment in working out problems.''

Discussing the ''dynamic of discontent,'' Hall declares:

> I for one, am grateful that times have changed. I still remember vividly the apathy of the unemployed in the early days of the depression. Relief was cut off for 10 weeks in Philadelphia while the legislature bickered as to appropriations. A study made at that time showed that many of the unemployed searched garbage pails for food. Just lately when the New Jersey legislature failed to make appropriations, the unemployed descended on the Capitol and settled down to make their plight

known; certainly for people brought up on ideas of democracy, a step ahead of searching garbage pails. It was encouraging that conservative papers carried this exploit with considerable sympathy and I did not happen to see the usual comment that the demonstrators must be Communists.

Hall reported the attacks on agencies, the threats, the withdrawal of support, but asserted:

We are by no means custodians of the whole truth; but there are some things we know close in and can share. Those of us who work with groups of young and old who are struggling and reaching out for opportunities learn that many of them bring to the struggle verve and initiative and courage to equal anything America has ever known.

That was 1936.

What about 1985?

In social work today in the United States settlement movement we do not have this regard for and this relationship to the poor. We are in contact with the poor, and we provide services for them, but in a different way — almost handling them with forceps in a sterile field — the human quality, the fraternal quality, of a common struggle is missing.

When we examine current proposals on what to do about the critical problems of youth unemployment, health care, the blatant as well as the more subtle racism in our society, the undercutting of welfare standards, etc., what do we find? Passive proposals for measures to dissipate apathy; to examine the problems; to reveal and interpret the facts; to clarify and highlight needs. All this is fine and needs doing, but if we stop at this point at knowing, and do not accept responsibility for doing, for acting, then we add to the despair.

The problems of minorities, the welfare family, the aged and the ill are social problems which cannot be solved piecemeal in each family. They necessitate social answers. The dynamics of discontent, where it is not socially organized, can sputter into jail sentences for stealing food and breaking the law in the countless ways the poor learn. Or it can short out the electric functioning of the human being and send him into the protective exile of mental breakdown. Many of them now live in the Single Room Occupancy hotels of my neighborhood. How true is this in your part of the world?

What is our role today in the feverish, disquieted world of change, where wealth trembles and glistens in the show windows, but where the poor cost too much, and the aged are all an encumbrance and health care is too expensive for too many of our neighbors?

Is it our role to teach the poor how to live quietly on less than minimum standards of health and decency and how to starve on the minimum wage? Do we teach them how to budget malnutrition more neatly? Or is it our job to struggle for those minimum standards, to cry out against the torment of the present and the annihilated future of the children? Or is it our job to involve our neighbors in their own struggle and to provide community leadership where we are — in the settlements?

If not, what are we saying? That social workers may speak for the poor with grace and decorum, presenting their plight and asking for ameliorative measures? They must not, however, on pain of excommunication from their funding sources help the poor, the unemployed, the old people, the deprived to speak for themselves.

We hear much of the hard-to-reach families in the low income groups, and they exist, and some of them are hard to reach. But there is another, larger group, multi-problem for sure, who are not hard to reach, who are unaffiliated because no one wants to affiliate with them, when push comes to shove, no one wants them to affiliate with each other. They are multi-problem families — they suffer from all the unsolved problems of our time — the problems of unequal education, the problems of our economy, the problems of the single parent family headed mostly by women, of automation and unemployment and the unequal distribution of the goods and services of our world, the problems of racist discrimination against and segregation of minorities, the problems of handicapping illness and old age, the problems of the unused and fermenting energies of the young who roll in breakers on the beachheads of unemployment. They are multi-problem but they are not hard to reach. When leadership is offered they affiliate. Leadership which accepts these families and their life experiences permits the development and growth of leadership out of the families themselves. The Social Group work process can free the powers of each person and connect the individual to the others and to the rest of life.

Thus when you work with oppressed people you cannot work with people and hide them at the same time. One thing they all recognize out of their life experience is a phony.

To engage openly in social action brings us full tilt to the problem of reprisal. It is not a new one for us.

To place the solving of the problems of the poor in today's world and the prevention of war and nuclear holocaust as crucial questions for social action in the settlements is this one-sided?

In order to solve crucial problems, it is necessary to choose crucial factors, to isolate the nub. When we speak of unemployment, functional illiteracy and the inequities of our world, of whom do we speak? It is the lowest fifth of our economic order. Where are the sharpest problems, the problems of no work at all or the empty succession of odd-jobs scrounged out of the garbage pails of our economy or the fierce competition for the unskilled and underpaid job in all areas of the world.

Let me tell you a story Jane Addams used to tell which she heard from Tolstoy:

> In Russia there is a sect of Doukhobors, a religious sect who do not believe in going to war. They are like the Quakers. When the young men become of military age and refuse to serve, they are arrested, punished, sometimes exiled or executed. One of the young men was brought before a humane judge, who felt sorry for him. The judge told him that he was very foolish to put himself up against a powerful government. The young man gave the judge a homily upon the teachings of Jesus in regard to non-resistance and the judge, being Russian Orthodox, said, "Of course, we all believe in that, but the time has not come to put it into practice." The young man answered, "The time may not have come for you, your honor, but the time has come for me."

The time may not have come for others, but I think the time has come for us as social workers who work with groups.

Group Services for the Hard to Reach in a New Age Settlement House

James Forte

SUMMARY. Group work provides a method of choice in serving the chronically mentally ill adults who have "fallen through the cracks" and found themselves lost and confused in large urban centers. This paper describes the work of the Daily Planet, a new age settlement house, serving this chronically mentally ill population. Consideration is given to the roots of its innovative group services program, its basic principles, and its comprehensive group services program and innovations in the view of the worker, the view of the group and the view of the member.

Over the last 15 years, thousands of chronically mentally ill adults, who were discharged from state mental hospitals, have flocked to large urban centers. Unskilled and demoralized by years in the institution, these adults struggle to survive, let alone live a life of dignity. Society, they feel, has abandoned them. The message from state and local leaders, business men and women, even human service providers, seems to say: "Obviously, they can't make it in the community. Send them back to the hospitals," or

James Forte is Group Work Services Coordinator at Richmond Community Diversion Incentive Program, Richmond, Virginia.

"Sure, they need help, but not in *my* neighborhood!" It is time for the human service providers to take the lead. This paper describes an agency which has striven to do this.

The Daily Planet, a small alternative settlement house, has achieved the miraculous in its work with the chronically mentally ill adults and others who have "fallen through the cracks." It has survived for 15 years and has developed a unique and effective group oriented approach to work with hard-to-reach populations. This paper examines their approach, its basic principles, and its blend of concepts and skills, common to traditional mainstream group work with innovations flavored by a distinctive New Age sensibility.

THE DAILY PLANET AND THE CHRONICALLY MENTALLY ILL

Richmond Jewish Family Services created the Daily Planet in 1971 as a outreach program designed to provide a crash pad and informal counseling (rap) service for teenagers who had problems stemming from dropping out and turning on. It was a small and flexible agency which developed a tradition of tending to the needs of those ignored by the rest of the community. Then from 1975 to 1984, the Daily Planet focused its attention primarily on the chronically mentally ill adults, a population which included some of the burnouts of the 60s. During this period the agency staff created a model approach.

The Planet is located in a fringe neighborhood; notorious as a ghetto for the mentally ill. Adult homes, boarding houses, and low rent apartment houses spill over with the rejects of Richmond, Virginia. Situated in an old house and supported by Social Work faculty from Virginia Commonwealth University along with Richmond human service providers, the Daily Planet has had a good foundation for its growth on the leading edge of area social services. Moreover, the cultural climate supports experimentation and the Planet staff has a deep pool of traditions from which to draw in forging its identity.

Many of these adults have been burned by the system and will not let that happen again. Services have been offered in cold, bureaucratic settings; in ways that threaten already fragile self-esteem; by staff who have preferred work with the "worried well" or have felt endangered by their clients; and through modalities such as medication and long term psychotherapy deemed useless by the chronically mentally ill adults.

The new age spirit embodies possibility and responsibility. Imbued with this spirit, Planet staff, consisting of young recent graduates from social work schools and non-professionals numbering between 6 and 12 depending on funding, has brought a new attitude towards their work. This attitude involves a constellation of ethics and values (Satin, 1978) such as the importance of self-development and service to others as an ideal means of personal growth, and values, such as diversity, quality, experimentation, mutual criticism and creativity. There is hope that perhaps the staff can convert the chronically mentally ill adults, waste products of our competitive industrial society, into useful contributors. This is accomplished by a dual focus on self-reliance and collective effort. The attitude becomes an invitation. "We know what it's like to be outside of society. Stop in, we guarantee that you won't be hassled. In fact, maybe we can help you or you can help us. If you like what you see, join in. If not, that's cool, too."

External conditions have fostered this attitude. Our economic marginality has been a blessing, not a threat-encouraging resourcefulness and giving us the freedom to do our own thing. Definite opposition from the mental health establishment has strengthened our resolve while contributing a clear notion of what we didn't want to do. Support from experienced professionals and involvement in the "mental health reform movement has increased our enthusiasm and conviction. With these conditions, the Planet works as a participatory organization welcoming the confused, the weak, and the alienated (Rothschild-Whitt, 1979).

BASIC PRINCIPLES

A set of guiding principles have emerged similar to the principles of other alternative and collective organizations which sprang up in the late 60s (Holleb & Abrahms, 1975). These principles guide staff and members in all agency operations as well as in the delivery of group services:

1. Distinctions between client and staff are minimized. While staff is bound by the role of helper, differences in role do not justify differences in status or power. All who enter the doors of the Planet relate on a common human level (Tropp, 1971).
2. Services are free or at a minimum cost.
3. As Planet staff time and energy should be spent in relating to, or directly helping members, excessive paperwork, politicizing, complying with organizational procedures or rules, and unnecessary meetings, should be avoided.
4. Professionals and clients alike are members of the Planet community with rights and responsibilities, with needs and strengths. Relationships are characterized by a mutuality which flows from this sense of community (Falck, 1984).
5. The Planet's physical and cultural environment shall meet the tastes of the users of the service — homelike, informal, casual, and sometimes even messy.
6. The timing and the rate of service usage is to be determined freely by agency members. Members are not expected to fit into structures like long term weekly therapy which might be uncomfortable.
7. The Daily Planet belongs to its members. Members are encouraged to participate in every facet of agency operation. They have a voice in the governance of the agency, joining in a consensual decision making process regarding agency policies, goals, and procedures.
8. Group is the modality of choice. One to one helping is a spin off from group work.
9. Every aspect of involvement in the agency from the least mundane to the most complex is considered to have therapeutic potential. Talking is not the only vehicle for growth. Picking up trash in front of the building or making sandwiches for hungry newcomers has value.

The above principles service as the ideal. They give coherence and purpose to staff interventions.

GROUP SERVICES AT THE DAILY PLANET

The Daily Planet group services program aims to provide experiences which would enable the chronically mentally ill to learn how to cope with the demands of life in the community. As creators of a new approach Planet staff previously believed that other practitioners of group work offered little and they preferred to learn from analysis of trial and error. However, upon reflection it appears that the works of several others show a kinship to our approach:

1. The socialization models of social work (McBroom, 1970; Hartford, 1971; Chilman, 1971) which are a planned attempt to socialize people who are undersocialized due to lengthy hospital stays.
2. The milieu therapy model of Cummings and Cummings (1962) reflect a clear and constant focus on the teaching of roles — friend, worker, receiver, giver and citizen.
3. The here and now reality orientation of earlier practitioners: Eisen, 1958; Kaplan, 1980; Lane, 1961; Jacobs, 1964, as seen in the Planet approach's humanistic conception of the worker and member.

THE DROP-IN LIVING ROOM PROGRAM

In the beginning, Jewish Family Services asked the clients and staff of its new crash pad to name the outreach center. A contest was held. The winning logo showed a phone book, the site for agency telephone counseling. The winning concept suggested that clients and staff, when answering the phone were transformed from Clark Kents into Supermen and Superwomen. The winning name was The Daily Planet with its ambitious statement of openness to and responsibility for the whole earth. In the naming process the commitment to collective effort and collective decision making was set.

All who have entered the doors to the agency in that old house on Grace Street immediately have experienced the living room program (described in greater detail by Segal & Baumohl, 1985). Called "a safe place in a hostile world" by a member, the Planet living room has functioned as a clearing house for survival information and survival services; as a conduit into a range of other group services; and as the physical location for much of agency milieu work. Members staff the intake desk where they orient newcomers and greet regulars. The 60 to 70 people who use the living room form a diverse cross section of society—predominantly the mentally ill. Guests also include students, neighbors, street people, retarded adults and alcoholics. Black and white, young and old, poor and not so poor, men and women, crazy and not so crazy, are expected to relate peacefully and do. The "Less than Ten Commandments," a set of rules developed over time by the members, help. More importantly, it is their place and it is a good place.

Members have the freedom to choose the level and timing of their participation in any of the group activities (listed on a bulletin board), in the work program (jobs listed on a chalk board) or in informal counseling. "Hanging out," reading a magazine, playing cards, sitting and staring into space are acceptable activities. Staff and regular members are confident that newcomers will at some time feel their interest aroused and become more involved in the agency life. Newcomers are assured by example as much as by word that they will not be forced or labeled or medicated or stigmatized while at the Daily Planet.

Staff know that newcomers have been feeling isolated and lacking a social support system. Network building becomes one of the most frequent activities in the living room (Maguire, 1980). Staff, students, and volunteers who mingle freely among the members regularly encourage the development of informal relationships which might evolve into helpful alliances. When someone faces a night sleeping in an alley garage, the word is put out—"Who can put Harry up for a couple of nights until he gets himself together?" As members identify other needs or problems, i.e., uncertainty about the effects of their medication, they are referred to peers with expertise in that matter. Friendships built on mutual help develop and continue.

Through the living room program, chronically mentally ill adults learn that they can become a part of the Daily Planet. If they accept this invitation, staff and/or other regular members review the terms of membership in an informal discussion. The discussions cover rules and basic expectations, members' needs and interests, and exploration of how the new member might contribute to the rest of the community. After entry, daily interaction provides many opportunities for education in the management of membership (Falck, 1984). Staff or peers might request an examination of interpersonal troubles ranging from the way one asks for cigarettes to exploitation of weaker members. This occurs warmly and openly at the moment of a troubling interaction. Onlookers are invited to help out. If a difficult situation recurs, it is referred to the community meeting.

Living room users form the pool of people who would be recruited for group services and Rainbow jobs. A leader makes the rounds — "It's time for community meeting in the next room. How about joining in?" or "We need another worker for the Marsh job. Who would like to earn some money and cut some grass?" Usually members respond positively.

At the weekly community meeting, chronically mentally ill adults struggle with the feeling that they are powerless and have no control over their lives. As Keefe (1984) points out this leads to alienation and blocked personal development. At the community meetings, members discover that they have a stake in the Daily Planet and that their voices will be heard. Here, the community focuses on the real problems which arise during collective endeavors. The group leader, with the assistance of senior members, chairs the 90 minute meeting. All members are invited and attendance ranges from 12 to 25. The leader helps the group develop an agenda based on their concerns, problems and complaints. Issues are discussed one by one. A senior member — one who will not be overwhelmed by the demands of leadership — has the option of chairing the group during consideration of his/her item. The group leader or the temporary member leader guides the group through a deliberation, decision, and action process. Whenever possible decisions are arrived at by consensus. Majority rule prevails when there is controversy.

At the community meeting members deal with a variety of issues such as: "Should the Daily Planet lend space to a human rights organization? What response shall the community make to a member who refuses to stop cursing loudly in the living room? What shall be the plans for an upcoming Halloween party? How shall we deal with complaints from merchants who assert that Planet clients harass their customers? What is to be considered in the hiring of a new staff person?

Each year the community has elected two representatives to the Planet Board of Directors who also serve as the client group leaders. An election committee is selected from the membership and this committee has functioned with minimal staff guidance. It organizes and monitors the entire electoral process which consists of campaigns, debates, voting, and the recognition ceremony. It makes regular reports at the weekly community meeting.

The weekly community meeting provides the basis for the development of social action groups in response to community issues. For example, neighborhood organizations sponsored legislation at the city level for the purpose of closing adult homes. Staff and members united, developed a plan, and brought 40 members to a City Council meeting. Several members spoke eloquently on behalf of the mentally ill. As a result legislation was defeated.

Through the leadership of a dynamic ex-patient, the community formed the Scarlet Letter Group. This group addressed state wide advocacy issues and successfully lobbied for seed money for the creation of a member employment business called the Rainbow Services. Through these services, members learn about power (Pinderhughes, 1983), building coalitions, and taking political action inside and outside the Daily Planet. What better preparation for the role of citizen in a society that attempts to withhold power from the chronically mentally ill?

RAINBOW WORK SERVICES

Rainbow, a name selected by the members, refers to the pot of gold which waits at the end of the rainbow. Rainbow is a member employment service specializing in janitorial, landscaping, and housecleaning work. Few chronically mentally ill have the opportunity to earn money and to gain a sense of self-esteem through work. In contrast to community oriented programs that emphasize individual transitional employment programs or job placement services, the Planet has developed a group oriented training program.

Any member of the Daily Planet is eligible for work through Rainbow. After an orientation and assessment of work skills, the member, who is now considered to be a worker, attends a weekly group meeting. The staff introduces the new workers, presents available jobs for the week, and assists the workers in job work crew selection. Work crews of 3 to 5 members function as a team with the twofold task of relating harmoniously and of completing the job to the customer's satisfaction.

Rainbow work is structured to maximize the likelihood of worker success. Each work crew has a supervisor who is a staff member or a senior worker. Prior to employment, workers receive training in learning job related skills. They also learn how to give and accept criticism, resolve conflicts, and relate to authority figures. This team approach enables workers to advance at their own pace. There is a place for the least capable who might handle the vacuuming and for the most capable who might independently supervise a large landscaping crew. The work environment is supportive, noncompetitive, and playful. Workers take pride in their work and gain a sense of independence as they earn spending money.

ACTIVITY AND COUNSELING GROUPS

The Daily Planet offers a comprehensive group activities program designed to develop intellectual, aesthetic, physical, spiritual, and social capacities. These include arts and crafts, talent shows, group games' night, and drama, guitar, yoga, meditation, and photography groups. Members and nonprofessionals from the neighborhood with the interest and talent are encouraged to lead activities. For example, a talented street person led a successful mime and clown group that gave a performance at the local crippled children's hospital.

The agency places a strong emphasis on field trips. Outings to museums, bowling alleys, and to parks give the deinstitutionalized a safe and pleasurable way to learn again how to behave in public and develop skills crucial for reintegration into the community.

Staff and clients participate side by side in many activities groups. The Planet Trotters, our basketball team, renowned on the mental health clubhouse circuit and coached by a United Way volunteer, includes members and staff.

A weekly Rap Group, run by staff and open to all members, is a program highlight. The Rap Group serves as a forum for the exploration of survival issues and common concerns related to deinstitutionalization. The leader asks the group to select a topic for the evening, and develops a discussion of different concerns, feelings and coping responses. The members are viewed as the experts who have gained wisdom and know-how through their life experiences. Topics are wide ranging such as facing stigma as a mental patient; problems in receiving welfare benefits; tricks useful in obtaining food and shelter; values and hazards of psychotropic medications; feelings of loneliness; and detecting rip-off artists.

The leader makes a special effort to model sensitive and attentive listening to the mentally ill members and encourage the group to remain reality based. For example, a discussion on attending local church services could otherwise become too easily a philosophical debate between two members who each claimed status as representatives of God. The members' life experiences and their street/marginal lifestyle requires that the leader avoids making value judgements and tries to understand where each person is coming from.

LINKAGES BETWEEN INDIVIDUAL AND GROUP SERVICES

Planet staff values one to one helping efforts and encourages a natural flow between group and individual service. If a member in the drop-in living room, or on a Rainbow job, or at a group meeting reveals a need for special attention, the group leader would involve the agency caseworker. The caseworker, acting in conjunction with the group leader, works with the member and determines the need for other services. On the other hand, the caseworker and staff frequently refer clients to groups. This flow between group and individual services is beneficial in engaging hard to reach clients previously turned off to a particular helping method and has been responsible for the Planet's success in providing aid for those who would previously have required rehospitalization.

STAFF MEETINGS

The staff meeting is the place where it all happens. Staff meetings occur weekly and usually last for an hour and a half. Members are invited to one open staff meeting per month at which time they can present grievances or raise questions. Staff meetings follow a basic format: sharing of information regarding developments in agency, staff, or member life; formulation and discussion of agenda items relevant to goals, policies, and procedures, and exploration of practice problems.

Staff operations differ from the traditional team approach (Brill, 1976) in several innovative ways:

1. The agency administrator governs by consensus not fiat. Decisions about all aspects of the Planet are made through the use of the group process. Staff is accountable for their performance to the group as a whole rather than to administration. The administrator's function is to help everyone feel a part of the agency and to help the different groups operating within the agency relate harmoniously with each other and with the organization (Trecker, 1980).

2. Staff roles at the Planet are mainly interchangeable. Specialization is avoided. When a group leader is absent, another staff member would replace that person. When the director is on vacation, his responsibilities are delegated to various staff. This practice recognizes and encourages the development of individual strengths and promotes a sharing of responsibility.

3. All agency matters are open for consideration by staff. This includes: budget setting, grant writing, agency evaluation, hiring new staff, and policy changes.

4. Staff, students, and volunteers are expected to participate in group work training and to develop competence in the practice of group work. The agency provides group supervision to its group leaders.

The group approach with Planet staff engenders a strong commitment to the agency mission, insures the quality of agency services, dramatically lessens the burnout factor common to those who work with the chronically mentally ill.

CONCLUSION

When everything works as we dream it can, it is a marvel to behold. The Daily Planet has achieved some peaks of group performance and vitality. One group venture stands out. For two years in a row, the agency sponsored fund raising dinners for our constituents and friends. In 1983, the theme was "Buddy, can you spare a dime?" In 1984, the theme was "Big Brother is not watching." Board, staff, students, clients and friends have joined in planning these extravaganzas, attended each year by more than 200 people, and each year offered to the guests an incomparable meal, a guest speaker (the State Commissioner of Mental Health in 1983), fashion show, entertainment, and a comedy auction. At each, a good time was had by all. The spirit of community and teamwork spread like wildfire. The Planet's way of working with the chronically mentally ill and its claim to fame became manifest for all to see and feel.

The model does not answer all the questions. Unresolved issues remain: are there limits to consumer empowerment? How does a New Age type organization retain its identity in a time of tight funding and pressures toward conformity? What are the nuances of serving as a professional in a human and authentic fashion?

The Planet's model is not immune to threatened pressures to return to a traditional hierarchical structure where the bosses hold all the power. Pressures to retake the status, distance, and role protection which some professionals have come to prefer and pressures to regress to the days of mediocrity and indifference are still with us.

For those service providers who resist these pressures and who feel brave enough to innovate, the Daily Planet in Richmond, Virginia has demonstrated that a blend of the old with the new in social group work will enable the chronically mentally ill to find their place in the sun. In the words of rock poet, Elvis Costello, "What's so funny about peace, love, and understanding, anyhow?"

REFERENCES

Borkman, T. (1976). Experiential knowledge: A new concept for the analysis of self-help groups. *Social Service Review*, 50(3), 445-455.

Breton, M. (1984). A drop-in program for transient women: Promoting competence through the environment. *Social Work*, 29(6), 541-546.

Brill, N. (1976). Teamwork: Working together in the human services. Philadelphia: J. P. Lippincott Company.

Capser, M. (1981). The short term group: A special case in social work. Third Annual Symposium on the Advancement of Social Work with Groups (mimeo).

Chamberlin, J. (1978). On our own: Patient-controlled alternatives to the mental health system. New York: McGraw-Hill.

Chilman, C. (1971). Socialization and interpersonal change. *Encyclopedia of Social Work*, 2, 1295-1310.

Cummings, J. E. (1962). Ego and milieu: Theory and practice of environmental therapy. Chicago: Aldine.

Eisen, A. (1958). Group work with newly arrived patients in a mental hospital. *Social Work With Groups*, 94-105.

Falck, H. (1984). The membership model of social work. *Social Work*, 29(2), 155-160.

Gartner, A. (1976). Self-help and mental health. *Social Policy*, Sept/Oct., 28-47.

Hartford, M. (1971). Socialization methods in social work practice. *Encyclopedia of Social Work*, 2, 1311-1315.

Holleb, G. & Abrahms, W. (1975). Alternative in community mental health. Boston: Beacon Press.

Hoover, K., Raulinaitis, V. & Spaner, F. (1965). Therapeutic democracy: Group process as a corrective emotional experience. *International Journal of Social Psychiatry*, 2, 26-36.

Jacobs, J. (1964). Social action as therapy in a mental hospital. *Social Work*, 9(1), 54-61.

Jones, M. (1968). Beyond the therapeutic community. New Haven: Yale University Press.

Kaplan, I. (1960). Some aspects of group work in a psychiatric setting. *Social Work*, 5(3), 84-90.

Keefe, T. (1964). Alienation and social work practice. *Social Casework*, 65(3), 145-153.

Lane, D. (1961). Psychiatric patients learn a new way of life. *New Perspectives on Services to Groups*, 14-23.

Maguire, L. (1983). The interface of social workers with personal networks. *Social Work with Groups*, 3(3), 39-48.

McBroom, E. (1970). Socialization and social casework in R. Roberts & R. Nee, Theories of social casework. Chicago: University of Chicago Press, 315-351.

McCreath, J. (1984). New generation of chronic psychiatric patients. *Social Work*, 29(5), 436-441.

Pinderhughes, E. (1983). Empowerment for our clients and for ourselves. *Social Casework*, 64(6), 331-338.
Rothschild-Whitt, J. (1979). Making participatory organizations work in J. Case & R. Taylor (Eds.), Communes and collectives. New York: Pantheon, 215-244.
Satin, M. (1978). New age politics: Healing self and society. New York: Delta.
Schopler, J. & Galinsky, M. (1984). Meeting practice needs: Conceptualizing the open-ended group. *Social Work with Groups*, 7(2), 3-21.
Segal, S. & Baumohl, J. (1980). Engaging the disengaged: Proposals on madness and vagrancy. *Social Work*, 25(5), 358-365.
Segal, S. & Baumohl, J. (1981). Social work practice in community mental health. *Social Work*, 26(1), 16-24.
Segal, S. & Baumohl, J. (1985). The community living room. *Social Casework*, 66(2), 111-116.
Trecker, H. (1980). Administration as group process: Philosophy and concepts in Alissi, A., Perspectives on social group work practice: A book of readings. New York: The Free Press, 332-337.
Tropp, E. (1970). A methodology of group counseling in group work practice in a humanistic foundation for group work practice. Richmond: Virginia Commonwealth University Press, 218-228.
Tropp, E. (1976). A developmental theory in R. Roberts & H. Northern (Eds.), Theories of social work with groups. New York: Columbia University Press, 198-237.

Working with Families of Chronically Mentally Ill Individuals: A Psychoeducational Approach to Families Featuring Family and Professional Partnerships

Margaret Lazar

SUMMARY. The purpose of this article is to describe a particular psychoeducational group model for family members with a mentally ill relative. The model includes four specific outlines which address the different needs of parents, spouses, adult sibling and offspring, and teens. As well, a family member co-leads the group: he/she provides a link between the professionals and the client's families; the kind of working relationship needed between them is modelled.

It is well known that in the implementation of deinstitutionalization, the majority of psychiatric patients discharged from hospitals become the responsibility of family members. Lack of information regarding their relatives' illness and ways to deal with the problem associated with it, leaves family members fearful, confused and at times acting in ways that at best nullify, and at worst, sabotage treatment. This article describes a particular group model which attempts to address this problem.

A psychoeducational model, offered by Community Life Services, Inc., a community mental health center in Pennsylvania, provides the information needed by family members. Its unique features include four specific outlines which address the different

---

Margaret Lazar is associated with Community Life Services, Inc., Mental Health/Mental Retardation Programs, Sharon Hill, Pennsylvania.

needs of parents, spouses, adult sibling and offspring, and teens, and the use of a peer consultant as co-leader. The peer consultant is a trained family member of someone who is chronically mentally ill; as nonprofessionals, they provide a link between professionals and the client's families.

The process of deinstitutionalization has resulted in the need to maintain clients with chronic mental illness in the community rather than the hospital. Additionally, a whole new class of younger, newly diagnosed clients who have never been hospitalized, but are treated within the community mental health system, has emerged. For most of these two groups, the family has become the primary care giver; they "must cope with the practical consideration of caring for the psychiatric patient in the home. They must deal with feelings of entrapment and chronic overload, of role strain due to having to neglect their responsibilities to other family members, and of futility, confusion, isolation and exhaustion" (Thurer, 1983, 1162).

Treatment of these families has become an increasingly important issue. Theories in the past, which have been discredited, implicated family members in the development of the illness of their relative. The belief that parents cause schizophrenia in their offspring birthed a number of family therapy models: in attempting to change the family system to "cure" the mentally ill person, they met with little success. However, this type of family therapy has left families with a great deal of guilt.

By the early 1970s many therapists were becoming disillusioned with family therapy for schizophrenics (Leff, 1979). For example, Rubenstein (1974) writes "one of our earliest preconceptions, which proved to be unwarranted with the passage of time and our increase in experience, was that schizophrenic behavior could easily be modified if we treated the family conjointly, and if we helped the members sort our some of their interpersonal dynamics." Mental health professionals have begun to understand some of the neurophysiological and genetic components of the illness. While no longer believing the family caused the illness, they continue to believe the family maintains it. This is reflected in the language of the professional, families are "overmeshed," "overinvolved," or else, "cold and rejecting," "passive," and "resistant."

Thurner (1983) writes about the mother of an individual with a psychiatric illness.

> She is expected to oversee a treatment plan, no matter how unrealistic in terms of time, energy, money, and the demands of the rest of the family. She is expected to do so with little outside support, much conflicting advice from a variety of professionals, and with little promise of success. When things do not go smoothly, she is blamed. Should she discourage her child from unnecessary risks, she may be deemed overprotective. Should she encourage independence or seek residential placement, she may be deemed neglectful or rejecting. Should she demur from following any professional advice, she may be called a saboteur. (1163)

As a result many family members experience much anger at the mental health system which has ignored their input regarding their relatives' condition, and overlooked their concerns and questions. They experience a sense of powerlessness and hopelessness in maintaining any control over the situation. It is apparent that treatment of chronically mentally ill people must involve a joint partnership of both families and professionals. To enable this process to occur, families need to be given information regarding the illness and its home management and professionals need to acquire a respect for families' expertise in "treating" the illness.

In 1982, Community Life Services, Inc., a community mental health center in Pennsylvania, developed and implemented a psychoeducational group model which addresses these issues. Its goals are:

A. To provide information about mental illness and its symptoms; treatment options; resources available for clients and their families; and the structure and organization of the mental health system.

B. To teach family members how to communicate with someone who is mentally ill, how to approach problems they are facing with their relative, and how to plan for the future.

   C. To empower families through education, so that they are able to deal with crisis, including violence, suicide and noncompliance.

   D. To decrease families' sense of isolation by providing a group forum for members to receive support.

   E. To enable family members to get on with their own lives despite having a mentally ill relative.

This highly structured, supportive psychoeducational model differs markedly from a traditional therapeutic model. Rather than a group which encourages catharsis for its intrinsic benefit and uses spontaneous material from group members, this model provides a structured program with group leaders who act as educators and facilitators rather than therapists.

In line with the goals suggested by Anderson, Hogarty, and Reiss (1980) "The program seeks to increase the predictability and stability of the family environment by decreasing members' anxiety about the patient and increasing their self-confidence, knowledge about the illness, and ability to react constructively to the patient" (492). Practical how-to's are provided which increase members' sense of power and control over the situation, and decrease their sense of hopelessness and depression.

The model has a number of unique features:

Each group is co-led by a *peer consultant*; a trained family member of someone who is chronically mentally ill. This family member provides a bridge between professional and families, the kind of working relationship needed between them is modelled. Families have felt threatened by professionals; they have accepted decisions made about their relative, often involving them, without questions. For example, relatives often accept the patient from the hospital when they are so "incapacitated by the anxiety and strain" that they are "unable to cope with the disturbed member" (Anderson & Meisel, 1976, 868). They are expected to take care of their relatives with little or no information about their condition or progress. Also, professionals have disregarded valuable information from family members about their relative.

Use of the peer consultant provides validation to families that professionals respect their expertise. They, in turn, are able to help clarify issues to the professional from a family members' viewpoint. When group members begin to look at approaches to deal with the problems they are facing, the peer consultant is in a better position to challenge and confront group members' past methods of dealing with situations. She/he is able to nullify group members' defenses and encourage them to attempt things that were previously untried. Working with a professional, they provide a role model for group members of the working relationship needed between the professional and family. For family members, they also provide a sense of hope that there are ways to effectively deal with the overwhelming problems they experience.

When these groups began in 1982, they were run as a generic model. That is, all family members, no matter what their relationship to the client, attended together. It was found that although there are many issues and concerns that are generic for all population groups, each relative group experiences their problems in a different way. For example, parents are faced with the dilemma of separation from their mentally ill child in order for the child to become independent, while at the same time not abandoning them as they need support. Spouses, on the other hand, explore separation from a very different standpoint; their issues center around whether or not to stay in the marriage.

As a result, the workshop model has been tailored to serve four different population groups: parents, spouses, adult sibling and offspring, and teens. Some generic themes are addressed in each group series, as well as topics that are specific to that population group. These themes will be explored later in this article.

The groups are time limited; they run for ten sessions each at one and a half hours in length. It is well known in the group work literature that time limited groups encourage problem solving and facilitate a reduction in drop out rates. People who might reject services tend to remain in the group and work at the problems at hand. This closed group model also aids cohesion and trust between group members; a key ingredient to decrease isolation that family members experience living with a mentally ill relative.

ISSUES FOR RELATIVES

Family members attend these groups with a range of feelings which occur as a result of the process of coming to terms with mental illness in the family. Analogous to the bereavement process outlined by Kübler-Ross (1975) family members mourn the death of someone they once knew, and come to accept a stranger whose future is uncertain and whose behavior is unpredictable. "Initially, they may categorically refuse to accept the diagnosis, deny the illness and blame psychiatry on the one hand for 'labeling' and on the other hand for not curing their relative. This is often manifested as anger with the doctor and the institution. It may lead to frequent, frustrating attempts at finding the 'right' treatment."

Depression in the relative may be seen when the patient is acutely ill or when the potential duration of the illness and the need for long term treatment is finally realized. Acceptance of the need for treatment and support from relatives is potentially very valuable in terms of maintaining the patient's stability" (Thornton, Plummer, Seeman & Littman, 1981, p. 342). The group process facilitates members' movement away from any emotions they may be "stuck in" towards an end point where they are able to care for their mentally ill relative while caring for themselves at the same time.

Beginning Sessions

Initially, each group explores these feelings and their effect on decisions made about their relative. The group begins with a scenario involving a crisis situation for the family member; participants are asked to describe how this parent, spouse, or sibling may feel. Options to deal with the crisis are explored and group members begin to look at how their emotions affect their decisions. For example, a relative who feels angry about a situation may respond differently from someone who is anxious. Decision conflicts are explored. Parents discuss the conflicts which emerge when each parent makes a different decision about a problem with their child. Spouses, on the other hand, examine their ideas of how a "good" spouse would respond and how this conflicts with what they may prefer to do. Sons and daughters also look at society's view of what "good" children "should" do. The aid of this process, which takes a number of sessions, is to enable family members to make decisions which involve their "thinking," "decision making" parts as well as responding to emotional reactions. Permission is given to experience the range of feelings mentioned previously; however, participants are encouraged not to be directed by these.

Throughout these sessions, information is given about chronic mental illness and its characteristics. Inability to deal with stress and change, dependency on others, and inability to maintain mutually satisfying intimate relationships are the features which are emphasized. Schizophrenia, bi-polar illness, other affective disorders, and personality disorders are the illnesses which are described. The DSM III manual and diagnosis is explained, as well as information about etiology, symptoms and treatment. At this point, hereditary issues emerge for relatives: parents and spouses question the possibility of their children inheriting the disease; and sibling and offspring are concerned about their own susceptibility to the illness.

It has been documented that "education regarding illness decreases the likelihood of negative or oversimplified views of the patient" (Anderson, Hogarty & Reiss, 1980, 493). Family members come to accept that their mentally ill relative is not just lazy; nor does she/he have any control over their behavior.

Middle Sessions

The groups then begin to problem solve; a specific model which is used to approach problems is described, and family members implement the model. The rationale for planning prior to a crisis occurring is explained; members look at specific problems they are experiencing and the group brainstorms options for each member's problems. Specific techniques for problems such as violence and suicide are given.

Family members come up with a range of problems. Mental illness "presents features such as withdrawal, confusing communications, and unpredictable behaviors that are likely to make family life difficult. In general, the family is encouraged to set limits on unreasonable and bizarre behavior, and to do so before the tension builds, others become upset and a blow-up occurs. Overall, the family is encouraged to normalize their routine and interaction as much as is possible, and not to keep waiting for the patient's 'other shoe to drop' " (Anderson et al., 493).

"Relatives can be helped to see that it is often useless to contradict delusional ideas, but that patients can be told not to talk back to hallucinations in public. They can also be helped to understand that social withdrawal may be a necessary defense for schizophrenics, but that too much withdrawal may lead to a form of institutionalism at home" (Lamb & Oliphante, 1978, 805).

Limit setting techniques, which include behavior modification principles, are taught. Throughout these sessions, relatives are faced with a number of different issues. Parents are confronted with the necessity of encouraging independence in their children; this may cause a resurfacing of feelings of guilt and responsibility. Spouses begin to realize that the mental illness has forced permanent changes in their relationship which "prevents the shared intimacies that contribute to a marriage" (Bernheim, Levine & Beale, 1982, 168). This realization results in a great deal of sadness, and spouses may begin to seriously question whether or not they want to remain in the marriage. The degree of limit setting needed for sibling and offspring depends very much on whether the mentally ill relative lives with them or not. Offspring commonly express anger and sadness over their loss of childhood and their needs to take on a parenting role with their parents.

The groups then move on to explore communication techniques with someone who is mentally ill. A role play is enacted which illustrates for group members an explanation of auditory hallucinations. As a result of this role play, members take on the role of a person with mental illness so that they can understand some of the difficulties they have communicating. Members, as a result of exploring their own feelings, are able to begin to examine what it is like for their relative. Communication skills are taught, with explanations of client's need for withdrawal and low levels of stimuli, as well as the concept of expressed emotion (Platman, 921-925; Falloon, Boyd & McGill, 1984). Through role play, members are able to look at ways of communicating which lower their expressed emotion. Specific techniques instruct relatives as to how to give positive reinforcement and constructive criticism.

Ending Sessions

Support networks and how to look into them are explored; members are given encouragement to decrease their isolation. Many relatives are exhausted by the practical tasks involved in caring for a mentally ill relative; often they carry out the role alone. For single parents and spouses, this becomes a particularly important factor; specific stress management techniques are taught.

The groups end with relatives examining the prognosis of their mentally ill relative. The dilemma for relatives is there is hope vs. despair and relatives are encouraged to keep their expectations realistic by not comparing their relative with others. For each population group there are concerns peculiar to them. Spousal issues commonly revolve around the marriage and child rearing. For them mental illness has effected a role change; often they become both breadwinner and single parent without the benefits of divorce. Bernheim (1982) writes: "the upshot of all these losses: intimate confidant, co-worker in the household, and income—is to undermine your sense of partnership in the marriage. Disruption of the usual sexual relationship often accompanies mental disability. This disruption is especially frequent during the early acute stages of the disorder." Group members discuss the effects of medication on sexual performance as well as the effect the illness has on the well spouse's sexual attraction to ill spouse.

Concerns also center around the effect the illness has on their children. Questions are discussed about hereditary issues; how to explain to their children about the illness; and what to do if children begin to have behavioral problems. Sibling and offspring are facing future caretaking decisions; often their parents have been caring for their mentally ill relative. The time is coming when they can no longer do that, and the sibling or offspring may need to take over.

Parents primary issue revolves around separation: while other adult children are now independent, the mentally ill son or daughter is still dependent, both financially and emotionally, on their parents for support. Parents need to face the separation issue so that their children can be independent, while still providing support so that they can function in the community.

GROUP LEADERSHIP

As mentioned previously, the leaders' prime task functions are as educators and facilitators. Although the group experience is "therapeutic" for group members; leaders do not act as therapists per se. Leadership is directive; group leaders select activities and interactions for a session only as they relate to specific goals. Any catharsis is goal-directed; emotions such as guilt and anxiety are examined in the light of their effect on behavior and decisions made. Decisions are encouraged which include the information received rather than being more reactions to an emotion.

The professional needs to switch his/her advocacy from the client to the family member in order to join with the group. Approaches to specific problems, such as dealing with a violent son, are examined in the light of the families' needs. It is hoped that any solution implemented will be beneficial for the client as well; however, this remains a secondary aim. Family members attend the group without their mentally ill relative; they are working out solutions for their problems rather than for their relatives.

Professionals also need to approach the group with an attitude of openness and honesty with information. Words like "chronic," "schizophrenia," "tardive," "dyskinesia" are important if relatives are to come to terms with the mental illness in the family.

GROUP PROCESS

Although not a therapeutic model, each group is seen to move through a process which parallels the process of acceptance of the illness.

A. Group formation and orientation of members: Here, recruitment of members occurs, using the peer consultant to invite potential members after an initial screening. Group goals are set early; as well, expectations are set up for what will happen in the group.

B. Conflict State: At this stage, members begin to accept their own position as relatives. Part of this process involves them examining their appropriateness for group membership;

many families see other group members as having relatives who are sicker, while theirs are "really not that bad." Here, one sees expressions of anger and members vying for attention in the group.

C. Maintenance Phase: This is a period of growth where norms operate smoothly. Members join with group supports and determine a course of action (they engage in problem solving). As personal issues begin to be resolved, group members are able to "switch over" and begin to understand what it's like for their mentally ill relative.

D. Termination Phase: Here, participants come to an acceptance of the illness. Sometimes, this takes more than a ten week series; relatives may attend a number of series or join an extended group which explores these issues in more detail.

Participants' evaluations of the workshops have been overwhelmingly positive. Among the ways they report being helped include: a greater understanding of their relative's illness, an increase in their ability to cope with situations that arise concerning their relative's illness, support from others and an increased understanding of themselves.

REFERENCES

Anderson, C. & Meisel, S. (1976). An assessment of family reaction to the stress of psychiatric illness. *Hospital and Community Psychiatry*, 27(12), p. 868.

Anders, C., Hogarty, G. & Reiss, D. (1980). Family treatment of adult schizophrenic patients: A psychoeducational approach. *Schizophrenia Bulletin*, 6(3), pp. 492-497.

Bernheim, Kayla F., Levine, Richard & Beale, Caraline, T. (1982). *The caring family living with chronic mental illness*. New York: Random House, pp. 168-169.

Falloon, I. R., Boyd, J. L. & McGill, C. (1984). *Family care of schizophrenia*. New York: The Guilford Press.

Kübler-Ross, E. (1975). *Death: The Final Stage of Growth*. New Jersey: Prentice-Hall.

Lamb, H. R. & Oliphante, E. (1978). Schizophrenia through the eyes of families. *Hospitals and Community Psychiatry*, 29(12), p. 805.

Leff, J. (1979). Development in family treatment of schizophrenia. *Psychiatric Quarterly*, 51(3), Fall.

Platman, Stanley R. (198). *Family care of schizophrenia*. New York: The Guilford Press.

Rubenstein, D. (1974). Techniques in family psychotherapy of schizophrenia in Cancro, R., Fox, N. & Shapiro, L. E. (Eds)., *Strategic intervention in schizophrenia*. New York: Behavioral Publications.

Thornton, J. E., Plummer, E., Seeman, M. & Littman, S. (1981). Schizophrenia: Group support for relatives. *Canadian Journal of Psychiatry*, *26*, August.

Thurner, S. L. (1983). Deinstitutionalization and women: Where the buck stops. *Hospital and Community Psychiatry*, *34*(12), December, pp. 1162-1163.

Case Study of an Activity-Discussion Group for Mentally Ill Adults in Aftercare

Betty J. Hitchcock

SUMMARY. This paper will present a description of a group of mentally ill adults, designed to foster independence, improve socialization capacities, enhance self-esteem, and learn problem solving skills. The audience will be given background information for the project and will participate in activities used within the group.

It is a winter morning and the snow has been falling long enough to cover much of the grime and litter of the inner city. On the second floor of an old downtown church, the excited voices of nine men and women contrast with the silent storm. The snow is brilliant and provides light into the dim room. The group, however, is oblivious to the weather, even though they will soon have to take city buses back to their separate group homes. They are intently involved in a challenging exercise, to walk across the 2 × 8 boards at various heights from the floor. There is spontaneous laughter as they encourage each other, offering a steadying hand to those who feel unsure. They cheer and applaud when someone successfully "walks the plank." They are experiencing in a concrete way the stimulation of accomplishing a difficult task and the satisfaction of being part of another's success.

The spontaneous interactions and risk taking in this true scene were not typical behaviors for the eight group members, who like

Betty J. Hitchcock is a Practitioner in Hazel Park, Michigan.

many other chronic mentally ill adults in aftercare programs, tend to be withdrawn, socially inept and dependent. One of the challenges presented by aftercare services for mentally ill adults is to deal with the problematic behaviors of the most disturbed and still have time and energy to help clients who have the potential for integration into the community. Group work offers an efficient, effective, and exciting modality to meet the challenge. Realizing this, an occupational therapist and the writer, a graduate social work student, teamed together to design a group that would facilitate the transition into the community of their agency's higher functioning clients.

PLANNING STAGE

The six week planning period was used to select and recruit group members, define specific goals, design the format, and finalize logistics. The group was composed of eight adults whose common characteristic was chronicity of mental illness, each having had multiple hospitalizations and community placements. The primary selection criteria was that the person be currently involved in programming outside the group home, capable of independent travel, and demonstrated a capacity for increased independence and personal interactions. The selected group consisted of five men and three women, ranging in age from 26-55. One young woman walked with a prosthesis. Three of the men had problems with alcohol use. The group was diverse in degree of psychosis and socialization skills.

Once selected, each participant received a personal explanation and invitation to join the group, which was presented as special recognition of their efforts and an opportunity for them to be involved in an enjoyable support group. Some were skeptical that it could be anything but another gripe session. This was countered by the enthusiasm of the leader. "I don't like to be depressed either! We are planning an enjoyable experience for us all." Only one person declined to participate. Verbal commitments were made by the members to make an effort to attend each session.

The goals had to be carefully defined since they would influence every aspect of the group. The original and pervasive objectives were to recognize, encourage and facilitate the efforts of members to improve their lives and to integrate into the community. The specific goals to achieve this were to foster independence by improving problem solving skills, by expecting responsible, goal directed behavior, and by requiring autonomous decision making. The other major goal was to improve social and communication skills by providing a structure which would encourage both studied and spontaneous interactions.

In designing the format, the characteristics of the agency, leaders, and members were considered. An activity-discussion design was consistent with the behavioral approach of the agency, which stresses social functioning, not insight, as the treatment goal. Furthermore, the design fit especially well with the social worker's group orientation. Her enthusiasm for the approach reassured and energized the members in early sessions. The typically lethargic behavior of the majority of members was also considered. The planned exercise had to be stimulating, relevant, simple, non-threatening, and fun, combining team effort with an opportunity for individuals to learn, test, and practice new skills and perceptions. The exercises were planned to relate to the discussion topics as simulations of real life. While anticipating the interests of the members, the leaders consciously tried to remain flexible by regularly eliciting feedback from the members once the group began.

The logistics reflected the goals and external constraints upon the group. Because of time on the student social worker, the group was confined to eight, one-hour, weekly sessions. The group was to begin and end on time to foster time competency. Coffee, hot chocolate, and snacks would be available to early arrivers. Because members came from four different group homes by public transportation, it was necessary to find an accessible, central location with privacy and a room large enough for activities. A suitable church was selected because it had the added advantage of being a non-stigmatizing community resource.

From the first to last session, the levels of interaction, risk taking, and abstraction grew observably. This case study will focus on how both group process and the structured interactions fostered in-

dependence and self-esteem, as well as improved social and communication skills.

IMPLEMENTATION STAGE

The group evolved through identifiable stages of development:
forming, storming, norming and performing (Tuckman, 1965). We
added a fifth stage, reforming, in which the group evaluated itself.
The forming stage began the day before the first session. Each
member was called to remind them of the group and encourage
them to come. Only one member was absent the first session, and
this was the person the leaders had spent the least time recruiting.
Following the session, he was contacted by the leader and the group
was explained in more detail. He attended all the remaining sessions.

The first session was carefully planned to be a get acquainted,
orientation time, with a simple device to encourage discussion
about what the members wanted from the group. Members were
asked to complete this sentence with one word: I want the group to
be _____. The responses were written on a blackboard. Each
member was then asked to choose the most important word and to
tell why. The most psychotic and withdrawn member surprised the
leaders by saying, "I hope this group is fun. Every group I've ever
been in has been depressing. I think I could talk if I was having
fun." This was more verbiage than we had ever heard from him at
one time. The therapeutic value of humor became evident as the
group evolved.

The group began storming in Sessions Two when three of the
men came in late. Tardiness is a common form of resistance with
schizophrenics, as it is with other groups (Walker & McLeod,
1982). Their resistance was not confronted directly; instead, the
group started without them and was occupied in a stimulating activity when they came in. By Session Four, tardiness was no longer a
problem and attendance held at seven or eight for each session.

Norming was initiated in the first session by starting on time,
taking a light-hearted approach, and talking openly about what
leaders and members expected of each other. In Sessions Two and
Three, tardiness, pacing, interrupting, bumming cigarettes, and

rambling speech were identified as unacceptable behaviors. When these occurred, the leaders simply suggested that the behaviors hindered the group. By Session Five, these behaviors were minimal. On the positive side, everyone's opinion was valued, and no one was coerced to do anything against his will.

By Session Four, the group was performing. At the suggestion of the group, the topic was how to handle authority figures. The session was a game, *You're Hot!*,[1] to simulate the receiving of conflicting order from people. Members were then asked to tell of some problem they were having with a supervisor. Two situations were chosen and assigned to four members for role play. One group had a member sorting books. Two people came by and complimented him. The third, his supervisor, came by and told him it was wrong. Discussion followed. How did he react? How did he feel? Does he ever talk to the supervisor? Does he feel appreciated? How could he have handled the situation differently? The group had progressed to the point where they could collaborate on problem solving. The session ended five minutes late, with the leader saying, "Time's up! We've got to quit!"

The group continued to perform with increasing confidence and verbalization. In Session Five, they *Walked the Plank*.[2] By Session Seven they were able to choose peer guides to take them blindfolded through an indoor obstacle course.

The group entered the final stage, reforming, in Session Eight. After a game of *Whiffle Ball*, members evaluated the group with simple written forms and discussion. The leaders were impressed that members grappled with some of the same issues with which

---

[1]*You're Hot!*: One person leaves the room. The group chooses an item to be hot. Person must find the item by group saying hot, warm, cold, etc. After several turns, group picks two items in different parts of the room to simulate hearing conflicting messages.

[2]*Walking the Plank*: The goal is to be able to walk across the highest plank, or other reasonable height. A 2×8 board is placed on the ground. All walk across. Board is then placed on two bricks. Someone stands on one end so the board does not flip up. After all have walked across, set the board between two chairs. The highest level is between two tables. People walk beside the person on the board, holding their hand if needed. Use discretion. This is a tremendously exciting and affirming experience. If people choose not to walk across the highest level, they are still affirmed because they have set realistic goals for themselves.

they had to struggle. One of these was the constraint of time, which sometimes necessitated a choice between discussion around the knowledge and concepts (content) of the preceding activity or the self-discovery and feelings (affect) generated by it. The occupational therapist tended to put priority on content and the social worker tended toward affect.

During the discussion, one member said that the group needed "more chance to support each other, to talk over our particular situation." Jim, who in Session One had wanted the group to be fun, piggy-backed on the comment. "I have the same feeling. Maybe instead of so many games, we should get to know each other better. You know, get more personal." His criticism was a grand compliment! The structured interactions had brought Jim to the point where he was no longer so reliant on them.

Concurrent with group process, activities and discussion also contributed to the achievement of desired outcomes. Two dynamics, concreteness and humor, were especially important in enabling members to learn and grow. These dynamics can best be illustrated by examining one complete session in some detail. The topic for Session Six was of great concern to the members, Getting a Job. The occupational therapist thought it was important for the concept of partializing goals and tasks which was presented in the *Walking the Plank* exercise the previous week be reinforced. She was also concerned that the members practice looking at their individual situation in order to set realistic goals. These are very abstract ideas. The challenge was to concretize them in such a way that overall group objectives would be attained. The possibility of designing an exercise similar to *Walking the Plank* was considered, but it seemed unlikely that the same energy and excitement could be generated the second time around.

The idea finally came to make use of the idiomatic expressions of baseball: Can't get to first base, Struck out, Standing out in left field, Warming the bench, and so forth. Perhaps these could be used to help members think about where they are in relation to their goals. The group had demonstrated that they could make use of metaphors if they were kept simple. The key was to design an activity that would involve the members physically in a simulation game, from which they could move gradually into concept and personal application. The following is how that was done.

9:50 WHIFFLE BALL: When enough members arrived, they were recruited to help set up a diamond using paper plates in the multi-purpose room. Members joined in as they arrived. The purpose was to let them physically experience and remember the structure of baseball as a framework for later discussion. No scores were kept. Members had to field the ball in order to have a turn at bat. The play was awkward, but animated with much shouting and teasing. "Hey, Wally, you can't play first with your hands in your pocket! Here, here! Over here!" One member was absent with a sprained ankle. Everyone participated, even the woman with the prosthesis.

10:10 REFRESHMENTS: The group gathered around a table for apple juice and coffee. This provided a transition and time to settle down.

10:15 SETTING THE STAGE: The leader explained that just as we had used boards last week to talk about solving problems one step at a time, we would use baseball to think about getting a job. The leader displayed a poster with a diagram of a ball diamond, bleachers, bench, and batter's box. She asked members to identify each part.

10:20 ANALOGY: When we get serious about a job or any other goal, it's like saying "I want to play ball." Getting a job is not like playing on any sandlot team, but getting accepted on a sharp, competitive league team. Discuss until members have grasped the analogy.

10:25 BRAINSTORM: What are some of the things you would have to check out before you even tried out for such a team? The following answers were given by the members: Can you catch and hit? Can you get along with the coach? Can you get yourself there on time? Can you get a uniform? Can you be a team player, shag balls, etc.? The leader then pointed out that catching and hitting are skills necessary to play ball. Skills are needed to get a job also. She wrote "skills" after that item on the board. She then asked the members what getting along with the coach might mean in getting or holding a job. They connected the role of coach with the boss.

Each item was thus generalized to the skills and attitudes needed to get a job.

10:30 PERSONALIZE: Stickers with different sayings were placed on the table. Members were instructed to pick out one that said something about themselves. They were told to put their sticker on the diagram to illustrate where they think they are in reaching their goals. The leader gave an example. "If you are not doing anything to get in the game and you're just watching other people get their life together, you could put your sticker on the spectator stands." They were eager to do this, and lined up to wait their turn. The choice of stickers, placement and comments were generally appropriate. Jim, who has three different community involvements chose COPING and placed it in the bullpen. "I'm getting ready." Tim, who was just starting his first volunteer job, placed his sticker in left field. Larry placed his sticker on first base, saying "I'm just getting started." Jan, whose volunteer spot had just turned into part-time employment, placed a sunny face at the batter's box. "I made it to bat!"

10:45 APPLICATION: After everyone was seated and comments about the stickers were heard, their attention was refocused to the list on the blackboard. Question: If you had to choose one item to work on in order to get a job, get in the game, what would it be? Several responded that they needed better skills, and discussion turned to how to get the skills. One person said that he knew he had to start looking better. It was soon evident that if time had permitted, each one of these items would have sufficient material for a whole session.

10:57 CLOSING RITUAL: The leader explained, "I would like to teach you something special I have done with other groups. We are a close group, and I would like to close our meetings this way from now on." The *Circle Ritual* was practiced. Once we were holding hands in the circle, the leader asked, "Would anyone like to tell something you liked or learned today?" Comments were: "Whiffle Ball was fun! I'm learning to listen and understand. I need to be more helpful. I'm going to be nicer to people." They were told to squeeze the hand of the persons beside them before we turned outward, which they did. After the grunts and squeals of the twisting, two members gave an extra squeeze to another's hand.

DISCUSSION

The exercises and discussions of this session would not have been possible in earlier meetings, partly because of the development of group process, and partly because the leaders had to learn to keep the material concrete, which means simple, short, specific and stimulating. The extent of the member's concreteness was not fully understood until Sessions Two and Three, in which some of the activities were too difficult.

One illustration of keeping the activities simple, short, specific, and stimulating is in the use of the stickers. The procedure was kept simple by taking only one step at a time. Members chose and commented on their stickers before the next step, placing them on the diagram, was explained. Each step was short and manageable, since they had to choose only one sticker and one spot on the diagram. Although higher functioning persons might be able to talk about themselves in relation to the diagram without ever leaving their seats, these concrete thinkers were given a tool, a visible symbol, to manipulate as self-expression. The stickers also met the last criteria of stimulating. They were attractive, humorous novelties, which fostered interaction. Members leaned over the table, passing and reaching for stickers. "There is nothing so stimulating as people working together on a common project" (Boyd, 1971, p. 26).

The importance of the upbeat element of fun and humor was evident in several aspects of the group. During the storming stage, it made the group attractive to resisting members. They had been reassured by the leaders that the humor would never be at their expense. They grew to trust this promise enough by Session Seven to allow a peer guide to lead them, blind-folded, through an obstacle course. As described earlier, the therapeutic value of humor was vividly demonstrated in Jim's remarkable progress.

The ability to laugh at oneself and with others is an important social skill that members were able to practice in the group. In Session Two, members were asked to write a want ad listing the qualities they looked for in a friend. Tim, one of the young men who had come in late, worked intently on his ad. When the leader asked him if he was ready to read his, he grinned. "Wanted: Female friend. Pretty and fun. Must have a nice car." Everyone laughed. As the leader added his list of wants to the blackboard, she quipped, "You forgot rich!" More laughter. The next step was for them to write what qualities about themselves made them a good friend. They had more trouble with this than the first want ad. Tim wrote, "A good guy." The leader remarked, "It's a good thing you're not a rascal. We wouldn't want you taking advantage of that pretty girl with the car!" When it was time to dismiss, the latecomer's comment was "You mean it's over already?"

> Inoffensive, esteeming humor has been found consistently to increase the solidarity of group members. It acts as a social lubricant, easing group cohesion into a unified experience. Humor draws people closer together by relating to a common focus—the shared response to a single stimulus. In fact, the first signs of genuine laughter can sometimes be used as a yardstick to measure the progress of affiliative relations. (Kottler, 1983, p. 244)

Evaluation

Evaluation of the group was a continual process. After each session the leaders would debrief each other to identify what worked and what did not. Several midcourse corrections were made. The final session was planned for feedback and group closure. Consensus in that session was that the group was too short. The occupational therapist agreed, and subsequently reinstituted the group to meet during the Spring and Summer months.

Following Session Seven, a leader talked to Jan, a quiet 55-year-old woman, about the group. Her excerpted comments are an appropriate way to close this case study:

> I wasn't sure at first if I would like the group, but now I think about it at work and other times. I heard Larry telling someone about the boards and how it shows you can do things if you take one step at a time. I feel good and smile when I think about us getting up on those boards or playing ball. It (the group) encourages us to get serious about our goals. I'm talking to Sharon about getting my driver's license. We got so much into an hour. We are really into it, trying to figure out how to solve our problems, and it's time to go.

REFERENCES

Boyd, Neva (1971). *Play and game theory in group work.* Compiled by Paul Simon, University of Chicago Press, p. 26.

Kottler, Jeffrey (1983). *Pragmatic Group Leadership.* Monterey, California: Brooks Cole Publishing, p. 244.

Tuckman, B.W. (1965). Developmental sequences in small groups. *Psychological Bulletin* (63), p. 384-399.

Walker, John & McLeod, Gail. Group therapy with schizophrenics. *Social Work*, July, p. 364-366.

Friendship Camp:
A Model for Therapeutic
Summer Groupwork

Karl Weiland
Marty Zafran
Liza Brooks

SUMMARY. This paper describes the rationale for and operation of a therapeutic summer groupwork program designed for child and adolescent clients at a community mental health clinic. After providing a program description the authors discuss therapeutic aspects with reference to group development theory and activity choice, the holding environment, and the therapeutic nature of a recreational approach to summer groupwork.

INTRODUCTION

The purpose of this paper is to describe and discuss a model for therapeutic summer groupwork with children at a community mental health clinic. The model has been named "Friendship Camp," and has been implemented for four years by the Child and Adolescent Service (CAS) of the Somerville Mental Health Clinic (SMHC) in Somerville, Massachusetts.

Karl Weiland, Marty Zafran and Liza Brooks are Practitioners at the Somerville Mental Health Clinic, Somerville, Massachusetts.

Setting

The SMHC is a comprehensive community mental health clinic which serves the city of Somerville. Somerville is a densely populated, urban community which lies adjacent to Cambridge and across the Charles River from Boston. Somerville is a predominantly white, low-income community with a rich variety of neighborhoods and ethnic groups—Italian, Irish, Greek, Portuguese, Haitian, and Indo-Chinese. The CAS serves children from kindergarten through high school and their families.

Friendship Camp takes place at the main CAS location which is a one-time residential home converted into offices. There is a small yard adjacent to the building. In order to effectively implement the camp additional space was sought within the community. This has included a large playing field and an indoor gym.

Rationale

Friendship Camp was originally conceived to respond to a consistent seasonal difficulty of providing treatment services to children in the summer. Small-group therapy is suspended each June due to problems in maintaining attendance over the summer. Individual and family therapy continue, but are often interrupted by the vacation schedules of both clients and clinicians. In addition the suspension of school and hot weather generally mitigate against regular therapy contact. The day-camp concept is one that is familiar and acceptable to many children and families. CAS staff had consulted to community day camps for years and thus were aware that many CAS clients would not be accepted to or would not attend these community activities. It was decided, therefore, to create our own day-camp program which could be therapeutic and serve the CAS client population.

Friendship Camp was designed with two basic therapeutic purposes. First, it is a therapeutic experience for children whose regular treatment has been suspended or interrupted during the summer. Second, it performs a diagnostic function for new children. Areas such as developmental maturity, coordination, socialization, and ego-functioning can all be assessed within the context of the program.

PROGRAM DESCRIPTION

Population and Selection Process

As indicated above, the target population for Friendship Camp are the clients of the CAS. Children between 6 and 12 years old can be referred as "campers" by their primary therapists. The "core staff" of Friendship Camp, usually a group of 3-5 CAS staff, review the referrals and accept a group of 20. Selection criteria include age range and grouping, male/female ratio, management issues, perceived need, likelihood of attendance, and reason for referral, i.e., diagnostic vs. treatment considerations. Problem areas have included oppositional or disruptive behavior, academic problems, separation problems, victims of child abuse and incest, peer problems (both withdrawn and aggressive), eneuresis/encopresis, and disorders of mood.

Because the CAS includes adolescent clients for whom day camp would be inappropriate, the position of junior counselor was created. Adolescent clients between 14-17 years old can be referred for junior counselor positions at Friendship Camp. Once core staff person assumes the role of "j.c." coordinator. All referrals are interviewed and the core staff select 4-5 adolescents as paid jr. counselors. Selection criteria include male/female ratio, maturity, child care experience, work history, and perceived need, e.g., access to other work experiences. Problem areas have included depression, suicide attempts, drug and alcohol abuse, family conflict, and poor school performance.

Orientation and Training of Jr. Counselors

Once the j.c. group is selected an orientation meeting is held which begins the process of group-building. Policies and procedures of Camp are explained at the initial meeting which provides necessary information as well as a structure for member interaction. Questions and discussion are encouraged, food is supplied, and the identification of the group as the forum for support during camp is begun.

When camp begins j.c.s participate in daily pre and post camp planning and evaluation sessions. They are simultaneously considered part of the staff group and sub-group. Special time is devoted in sessions to their agenda which helps them structure boundaries for their roles and functions with "senior staff." The j.c. coordinator remains available to them for any concerns which cannot be addressed in the group, (although all j.c.s. have primary therapists at the Clinic as a junior counselor). The junior counselor experience is a perfect metaphor for the adolescents' position in their families and society. Their work in establishing appropriate roles and boundaries for themselves in Camp may be transferred to less supportive or more complicated settings.

Daily Activities

Friendship Camp is a program which runs three hours a day, three days a week, for two weeks in July. Although the theme of camp may vary each year and thus affect certain activities, there is a routine to each day which is consistent. We begin with greetings, songs, and orientation to the day's activity. The first activities involve more individual work, such as personalizing each camper's Camp tee-shirt, which is done in group context. Activities become more cooperative as each day goes on, so that structured interaction increases. While the first week of camp is usually devoted to activities which facilitate group development, the second week's activities are generally sequential in content and relate to the theme of the year.*

After completing the main activity of the day, the group returns to our base where a snack is shared and informal conversation about the day occurs. When it is time to end, campers and staff join together in a large circle. Any departures from the group, e.g., part-time staff who volunteered or campers unable to continue, are acknowledged and a long, loud "good-bye" is shouted to formally end the day together.

---

*The theme, for example, in 1984 was "Summer Olympics." Activities included making flags, parade ceremonies, and team games. The olympic games were presented as an example of international cooperation as well as competition, and issues of sameness and difference arose.

DISCUSSION

In this section we would like to discuss the therapeutic nature of Friendship Camp in relation to three concepts: (1) group process, development, and activity choice; (2) the holding environment; and (3) recreation as a therapeutic activity.

Group Process, Development and Activity Choice

Despite the brief life of the Friendship Camp group (2 weeks), the frequent and extended contact enables the group to progress through the stages of group development described by Garland, Jones and Kolodny (1976). Activities are incorporated in such a way as to reflect and facilitate group development. Such a short-term, structured, group approach to developing friendship skills has been reported by Lewis and Weinstein (1978) in use with small groups. The following is a description of various manifestations of group stages in the Camp program and activities which we have found useful in facilitation.

The first stage (pre-affiliation) is characterized by the silliness or shyness of new campers as they look around to see whom they know. Some campers stay with their mothers at the edge of the group as we begin our first morning circle. Siblings sit together and there is a clear focus on the staff and camp director. Name games are used to introduce each other. The camp songs are sung, which begins the campers' opportunity to master a body of common knowledge. The main activity for the first day is the distribution, decoration, and display of Camp tee-shirts. Campers receive one color; staff, including j.c.s, another color. For several days campers engage in non-competitive games. These activities serve to increase recognition, a sense of belonging, and initial trust within the group.

Stage two (power and control) in the Friendship Camp group is resolved in a different fashion than in smaller, therapeutic groups. Whereas small groups may be invited to participate in the planning and implementation of activities, Friendship Camp, by virtue of its size, heterogeneous ages, and time-limit requires a great deal of organization external to the group process itself. Broom and Selznick (1977) have described instrumental and expressive functions within a family or a group. The former function being one of planning and task orientation, while the latter is one of emotional relatedness. In this sense the staff perform most instrumental functions of the group separately, but maintain the expressive functions within the total group process. Since the group is already stratified (sr. counselors, jr. counselors, older campers, younger campers), members must achieve their status and role definition within boundaries which are more circumscribed than in smaller groups. However, perceived power is more diffusely distributed, i.e., among a number of senior and junior staff, so that campers may play out power issues with a variety of figures until they find a subgrouping which allows them a comfortable role. The great variety of activities and subgroups allows children of many types to gain positions of influence or achieve a degree of mastery. Dropout from camp is quite unusual and occurs primarily when a family goes away on vacations.

The working stages of intimacy and differentiation appear during the second week of camp. By this time a sense of belonging and clarification of relationships has been achieved. Camp songs are frequently sung or hummed spontaneously by campers. Parents report that some campers insist on daily washing of their tee-shirt so that it is ready each day, while other parents bemoan their children's insistence on keeping every grubby ribbon of valor on their shirt. Differentiation can be noted in that some campers choose to wear their regular clothes, which is usually accepted by the group without comment (in the first week questions are more common if a camper is not wearing the camp shirt). Activities involve more cooperation, e.g., team sports or games. Werner (1979) described from cross-cultural studies how peer socialization may lead to an affiliative rather than an achievement, i.e., competitive, orientation. The experience of belonging to a large, heterogeneous group and the use of non-competitive games encourages such affiliative socialization.

During these middle stages of the group the process of identification is quite active. What is so noteworthy about Friendship Camp are the multiple levels of identification. Jr. counselors and campers both imitate sr. counselors through dress and gesture. In addition, jr. counselors are able to use identification to practice new behaviors and roles in their relationships with each other and the campers. Of particular interest, however, are the identification processes which go on among campers and between campers and jr. counselors. Kolodny, Waldfogel and Burns (1960) noted that among the effects of camping as a therapeutic experience was the tendency for campers to admire jr. counselors and wish to have such a position. In Friendship Camp we have noticed the same phenomenon. This process of camper admiration of the jr. counselors is not only of potential benefit to the campers, but also results in a sense of heightened self-esteem, self-awareness, and responsibility on the part of the jr. counselors.

As with all time-limited interventions, separation is not a decision made through evolution, but rather one set in advance. Campers cope with the end of camp through anticipation and use of camp structures as well as personal defenses. The use of an "awards ceremony" in which each camper receives recognition for some contribution she/he has made to camp helps emphasize both individual strengths and their relationships to the group. Separation feelings are noted in campers who linger, act out, or withdraw at this time. Others manage by anticipating their involvement in camp the next year. It is noteworthy that campers do not react with avoidance; attendance is generally excellent throughout the duration of camp.

The Holding Environment

The holding environment is a concept derived from the work of Winnicott (1965). In his work this term refers to an interpersonal relationship between mother and child which supports the maturational process from dependence to relative independence of the child. Others have used different terms to describe this concept as it applies to groups. In considering the holding environment of small group psychotherapy Max Day (1963) spoke about the "therapeutic envelope." Maxwell Jones (1953) described the "therapeutic community," a holding environment concept which influenced the conceptualization of treatment in hospitals and residential settings.

The concept of the holding environment is a useful one in understanding the effect of Friendship Camp. By the end of the first week the boundary around the group and bonds within the group have developed such that there is a shared sense of togetherness which can support experimental behavior by some members as well as help those whose are struggling just to maintain their level of functioning.

The holding environment refers to the context in which campers establish relationships with one another. Although the activities of camp are structured to facilitate personal and social growth, many important contacts are made outside of the formal activities. This observation is similar to what those who work in residential treatment have reported. Bettleheim (1950) and Trieschman et al. (1969) have described the importance for psychosocial development of both structured and unstructured time in residential care and noted the usefulness of "life-space" interview in addition to those in office. At Friendship Camp it has been interesting to note intimate moments between campers or j.c.s. which occur at less focused times. During walks to and from the playing field children often pair up and may share thoughts or feelings about camp, themselves, or their families. Such connections are also made among children and between staff and campers during less-structured events such as snack or breaks during an activity. These "in-between times" offer both respite from the intensity of focused activities and casual opportunities to further intimacy. In a sense they are the glue which holds together the structure of camp.

Before leaving the notion of the holding environment we need to mention one important ingredient in its formation which Bettleheim and Trieschman have discussed. This is the use of routine and ritual. Routines in daily camp activities enable campers to make known comfortable people, places, and experiences which are at first unknown. Routines provide the security of knowing what comes next and how to do it. Rituals allow affects to be aroused and channeled through the use of symbolic experience. Our best example of this is the use of the "good-bye circle." The delicate matter of separation at the end of each day is handled by a ritual which is a part of the routine. The ritual heightens awareness of separation and then channels the expression of the aroused affect into a symbolic form of shared experience (circle, holding hands) and separation (shouting good-bye).*

Recreation as Therapeutic Activity

The use of activity, including non-verbal activities, as a group therapeutic approach with children has been established (Slavson & Schiffer, 1975). However, when the group is large and heterogeneous, moves from site to site, includes a variety of leaders, and meets for three hours daily, questions arise as to whether the evidence for small-group psychotherapy can apply to Friendship Camp. So far we have related the experience of Friendship Camp to models taken from small-group work (group dynamics) and residential treatment (the holding environment). In this final section we will briefly address the relationship between Friendship Camp and recreation, the model generally thought of for such large-group activities.

Recreation is generally considered an aspect of leisure time involving fun, relaxation, and playing. As such it is seen to be distinct from work, and to the extent that therapeutic activity is work, recreation is by definition not a therapeutic activity. Although such an opinion is not universally held, it is prevalent enough to frequently require justification of recreational activities in the service of mental health treatment. This occurs in the treatment of children, where recreational activities are more often used than in the treatment of adults.

The work of formulating the therapeutic nature of recreation is not new. One of the most interesting writers on this subject, and one whose work is here presented in relation to Friendship Camp, was Neva Boyd. In the early decades of this century, as she was training playground workers in social groupwork theory and practice, Neva Boyd made three points about the therapeutic nature of recreation (Simon, 1971): (1) that recreational activities can be used to enhance therapeutic group development; (2) that games can be used to

---

*This ritual was also used in a modified form, i.e., whispering instead of shouting, to say good-bye to the jr. counselor group in a separate meeting. The effect was quite powerful and led to a release of tearful feelings.

teach problem-solving skills, rather than as simply leisure activity; and (3) that emotional and cognitive changes can be achieved through physical activity. The first two points have been addressed in our previous section on group development and activity choice. The last point can perhaps be illustrated best by an example:

> Sally, a 10-year-old girl, arrived for camp in a skirt and well ironed blouse. Her parallel stiff and proper manner was partly an attempt to be a "good girl" and manage both rage and guilt left from an earlier history of victimization by sexual abuse. During an expressive activity with a professional clown Sally was able to put make-up on her nose and was soon swept up in the excitement of the group in nonverbal expression of various feelings. She eventually danced merrily with the clown and then joined the group in a loud good-bye. During the course of camp she dressed increasingly more informally. Her mother was first ambivalently, then pleasantly, surprised by changes she saw in Sally at home. Sally talked more with her mother and was eager to attend camp each day.

Obviously, not every child has such a dramatic response to camp. Also, no long term follow-up has been done to measure the lasting effect of changes. However, attendance to camp is generally excellent (93-97 percent average daily attendance), and parental feedback about enthusiasm and behavior change among children is not infrequent. There is a clear sense that we are providing an age-and seasonally-appropriate approach to engage these troubled children.

Sixty years has gone by since Neva Boyd began her writing on this subject. Society has changed; theories have changed; and the prevalence of various presenting problems in children has changed. Our experience at Friendship Camp, however, strongly confirms her observations and the conclusions she drew about the therapeutic nature of recreation. We have observed over 70 children in four years at Friendship Camp. With continuing effort we are learning how to incorporate activities into the natural process of group development with a large group in order to create a therapeutic outcome.

REFERENCES

Bettleheim, Bruno (1950). *Love Is Not Enough*. The Free Press: New York.

Broom, Leonard & Selznick, Philip (1977) (Eds.). Social status and social roles. In *Sociology: A Text with Adapted Readings*. New York: Harper & Row.

Day, Max (1963). The therapeutic envelope. Conference presentation, American Group Psychotherapy Assn.

Garland, James, Jones, Hubert & Kolodny, Ralph (1976). A model for stages of development in social work group, in *Explorations in Groupwork*, S. Bernstein, Ed., Boston, Mass.: Charles River Books.

Jones, Maxwell (1953). *The therapeutic community*. New York: Basic Books. Kolodny, Ralph, Waldfogel, Samuel & Burns, Virginia (1960). Summer camping in the treatment of ego-defective children. *Mental Hygiene*, 44:344-358.

Lewis, Karen & Weinstein, Lynn (1978). Friendship skills: Intense short-term intervention with latency-age children. *Social Work with Groups*, 1:179-286.

Simon, Paul, Ed. (1971). *Play and game theory in group work: Collected papers of Neva Boyd*. Chicago: University of Illinois Press.

Slavson, S.R. & Schiffer, Mortimer (1975). *Group psychotherapies for children*. New York: International University Press.

Trieschman, Albert, Whittaker, James & Brendtro, Larry (1969). *The other 23 hours*. Chicago: Aldine Company.

Werner, Emmy (1979). How children influence children: The role of peers in the socialization process. *Children Today*, 8:11-15.

Winnicott, Donald (1965). *The maturational process and the facilitating environment*. New York: International University Press.

Group Work in Industry

Claire Aschner

SUMMARY. This article explores group use in Employee Assistance Programs (EAPs). A brief outline of the development of EAPs, their function and objectives is included. The types of groups, their purpose and special considerations for group use in industry is discussed. The author concludes that groups are an effective component of EAP service delivery.

Industrial social work is one of the newer and most exciting forms of social work practice today. Programs sponsored by labor unions and corporations jointly aim to improve individual employee health and organizational productivity. This article is an attempt to explore how group work can be used to accomplish these goals. The type of groups, their purpose and the particular group dynamics found in the field of industrial social work will be outlined to provide background information. A rationale will be presented for implementing the regular use of groups targeted to the special needs of workers.

Social work in industry had its roots in the 1940s. Pioneers included Bertha Reynolds who established the first labor union program at the National Maritime Union, and Hyman Weiner who developed the Industrial Social Welfare Center at the Columbia University School of Social Work (9, p. 14). Programs were known primarily as Personal Service Units or Membership Assistance Programs in labor unions and Employee Assistance Programs or Employee Counseling Programs in corporations. The number of EAPs (the standard abbreviation for Employee Assistance Programs) has grown phenomenally over the last two decades, from 50 sites in

Claire Aschner is a practitioner at the Long Island Consultation Centers.

major corporations in 1959, to 300 in 1971, to 600 in 1973 and then to 2,500 in 1982 (17, p. 74). Deanna L. Thompson asserts that "more than 5,000 companies have initiated EAPs" (19, p. 40) and Bradley Googins, in a June 1985 article in the *Boston Chronicle* states that over 11,000 programs exist.

The tremendous growth in the number of EAPs can be attributed to four factors: organizational attitude, legislation, social and political change and escalating health care costs. Management and labor alike recognize that a worker's personal and family problems could be linked directly to losses in productivity expressed in increased absenteeism, lateness, accidents and a diminished capacity for performance. The most costly problems are caused by alcoholism and drug abuse with alcoholism alone accounting for an estimated $19.64 billion in lost production each year.[16,p.2] However, firing the dysfunctional worker creates new costs in the form of recruitment, hiring and training. Employee termination also creates poor morale and affects the public image of the organization. Sheila Akabas asserts that a more sophisticated management realizes that worker's personal problems "bite into productivity"[8,p.16] thus dispelling "the myth that family and work are separate worlds."[2,p.120] "Just as a person's work life may permeate other parts of his daily experience, so his troubles on the outside may be brought to the job. Worries and angers about relationships, debts and unmet needs, illness, about the care and safety of children—these and other concerns may so trouble the worker that job performance is seriously affected."[2,p.109] Social service assistance at the worksite is a logical, cost effective and humane response.

Federal legislation spurred the growth of industrial social work programs. The Civil Rights Acts of 1964 and 1965, the Alcohol Prevention and Treatment Act of 1970, the Equal Employment Opportunity Act of 1972 and the Vocational Rehabilitation Act of 1973 either provided incentives to organizations which established worker assistance programs or mandated that employees with special needs, mental and physical, not be discriminated against in hiring.

The last twenty years has seen a change in the composition of the U.S. labor force with increasing numbers of minorities and females (especially mothers of young children). Changing industrial needs created a huge pool of unemployed workers in need of retraining and social services. The longer lifespan, adding years of life post retirement (often with insufficient planning) targeted retirees as yet another group in need of service. A generation of women, traditionally available to care for aging relatives, were now members of the workforce and confronted by this role conflict. Women who left younger and younger children at home while they worked needed assistance in managing appropriate child care and in providing quality parenting.

Corporations and unions who provide health insurance as an employee benefit became concerned with escalating health care costs making cost containment an important consideration. ". . . Now a growing number of insurance companies and their corporate clients . . . are finding that they can lower overall health care costs by picking up the tab for psychotherapy, or by offering in-house mental health programs" (20, p. 12).

THE EAPs

An EAP has the following functions: to identify employees with problems through documented job performance criteria and to develop an appropriate course of treatment and rehabilitation so that the workers can retain their job and one hopes, improve their functioning.

Social workers were hired for EAP work because of their ability to work with individuals, to identify and understand outside stressors, to help people enhance their coping skills, to understand the organizational needs and objectives and to mediate between client and organization. Social workers were allowed into organizations but were not really welcomed. Barriers included pre-existing territoriality, especially from natural helpers who felt displaced; corporate doubts about the social worker's capacity to function in a product/profit world; misunderstanding of the helping process; and unreasonable supervisory demands and unrealistic expectations of the EAP.

The onus of establishing the EAP role is often left to the social worker. Successful clinical interventions and an ability to translate social work skills into the organization's language and culture help to convey the purpose of the EAP. Education of supervisors and employees about the counseling process, program policy (particularly confidentiality) and the use of groups can facilitate the integration of the EAP into the organization.

Although not a traditional area of practice, industrial social work can provide creative, responsive therapies, strategies for preventing mental health and even organizational change. But it can also be an area where the social worker is isolated and perceived with suspicion and mistrusted. Because group work can be used as a tool to further mutual support and to enhance individual and group functioning, the author proposes that groups can have a major role in industry.

In 1967, Hyman Weiner pointed out that "the union setting provides a fertile and potentially congenial setting for the practice of social work, and particularly for the utilization of the group approach."[1] In 1982, Kurzman and Akabas asserted that although ". . . clinical intervention is the most frequent method currently deployed in labor and management settings . . . excellent opportunities are available for group, community and administrative approaches"[2,p.215] Further, the same authors say that, ". . . Labor and management sponsored settings lend themselves to the use of self-help groups as a primary or secondary mode of intervention. Natural helping networks have been established around issues from weight loss to widowhood, from stress management to questions facing women in non-traditional occupations and titles."[2,p.216]

While these statements may allude to the value and use of groups in industrial sites, the literature of social group work is uninformative on the subject. Even within industrial social work little is written to document the extent of use, type, purpose and benefit derived from group work in these settings. One reason may be that social workers in industrial settings are not specifically trained group workers; they are either case workers or generalist practitioners. Several industrial student placements, including one union, will train only case work students because of the organization's emphasis on individual counseling.

THE STUDY

The lack of published material and the obvious value of group work in industrial settings warranted further exploration in this area. Therefore, the author developed the following two-phase study. Phase I consisted of a brief look at usage and types of groups as well as organizational obstacles in industrial settings. A literature review and interviews with practitioners formed the core of Phase I. Phase II is a research project designed to assess the extent to which groups are being used in industrial programs in the New York City area. The key questions included the number of employees served by each program, the number of program staff, the age of the program, whether groups were used (and if not, why), issues addressed by the groups, the frequency of meetings, purpose of the groups, background of the group leader, how group use has been evaluated and plans for expansion of this modality within the program.

Phase I Findings

The group format most commonly found in industrial settings is the one or two session seminar or workshop. Citibank, for example, has offered seminars on genetic counseling, marriage counseling, money management, adult relationships and parenting.[3,4] Banker's Trust is one of many corporations which hire independent consultants to present parenting seminars.[4] Hoffman-La Roch offers a weekly series on coping with divorce and separation.[5] Groups such as these offer participants the dual benefit of education and mutual support. One participant in a corporate parenting seminar said, "I think it's so helpful to realize you're not alone — to hear other parents talk."[5] Laboratory training groups, held off-site, provide an experiential opportunity for personal growth and enhanced problem solving through a small group setting.[6] Quality circles allow for problem solving and decision making to help participants improve work life and set and achieve goals.

Groups can be used effectively to help employees cope with stress and job satisfaction problems. For example, a group of workers in public welfare and child protective agencies found that, ". . . A small group approach, with its possibilities for collective group support, problem solving and sharing of personal and professional resources could be useful in helping staff to manage work stress more constructively"[7,p.57] In a labor setting, a joint group of mental health professionals and union business agents worked collaboratively to develop strategies to help the mentally impaired worker.[1]

Once they become accepted into the organizational culture, EAP workers can increase the use of groups in the area of prevention. Mount Sinai Hospital's EAP for instance, identifies high risk groups such as women workers who recently gave birth and runs ongoing groups for them. These groups focus on problem solving and concrete issues such as child care and transportation.[8,p.18] At Polaroid, workers who are assigned to a late shift use a group format to assess the effects of the shift change on themselves and their families. The group is empowered to determine when the late shift poses an irrevocable threat and can appeal for a reverse transfer.[8,p.17] When a hospital planned to move to a new wing, two half-day group workshops were offered to help the employees. "The feedback was very positive, with staff stating they were less anxious about the move and feeling more prepared to cope."[9,p.29] Groups have helped working parents manage their epileptic and mentally retarded children.[10]

To summarize, the research indicates that groups, mostly of limited frequency, do thrive in industry and do serve workers effectively. One could question the validity of the single session group in terms of group work theory and practice. Lawrence Shulman, while recognizing the validity of single session groups, recommends that material is presented both interactively and didactically to facilitate the participant's ability to absorb the information. A single session group can be viewed "as if it were a small group . . . by attempting to adapt the basic model to the group's limitation"[11,p.329] Shulman suggests that the developmental phases of a group can be conceptualized as condensed within the single session. Contracting is still valid, and members' expectations and perceived needs can be reached for in the first few minutes. The leader can then tailor the presentation with sensitivity to the group, resulting in greater participant attentiveness with the assurance of focus on each member's particular concerns. He concludes "that even a single session group with large numbers can be involved actively in a group process with beneficial results.''[11,p.31]

Confidentiality, leader training and criteria for group membership are the three critical factors in industrial group work. Confidentiality has a greater impact at the work site than in other traditional social work settings where groups are found. The worker's connection to the employing organization is complicated. At a mental health center, for example, a group member can decide to terminate after a perceived or real threat to confidentiality. But such a decision in a work site group would have deeper consequences. In addition, at work, group members may be unable to avoid interacting outside of the group. Thus, they may be reluctant to become involved in a group or maybe resistant to self disclosure. It is essential that confidentiality be handled seriously and sensitively. Helpful strategies include asking members to "sign a contract between themselves and the therapist pledging confidentiality" and ". . . to have all group members declared agents of the therapist and bring them under existing privileged communication statutes.''[12,p.134]

As in all groups, leaders in industrial settings should be professionals well trained in group process. They must be comfortable with limitations on personal disclosure, realistic about the frequency that workers can attend groups and flexible about the time demands of potential members' work lives. For example, the lunch hour may be the only time available to working parents as their personal obligations may preclude coming to work earlier or staying late; several workers in the same small department may be unable to attend the same group as they may be required to cover for each other during lunch.

Furthermore, worker relationships with respect to status may be an important factor in group composition. For example, if the topic is stress and if the employee's role and work site relationships increase that stress, it may be necessary to distinguish between the stress in supervising and the stress in being supervised. Being in a group with one's boss just doesn't work! Even in groups for "the working parents," a clock punching clerical mother and a fast track executive mother may have such different problems and options that it is impossible to develop mutual support so necessary for effective group work. When addressing such topics as fitness, nutrition and caring for an aging relative, status issues may be less relevant.

Phase II: Method and Findings

The data were gathered from responses to a letter and questionnaire. Management sponsored EAPs were targeted, but hospital, government agency, and union based programs were included. Corporate EAPs were to be more closely scrutinized because the author hypothesized that group utilization is more compatible with union philosophy. "The trade union, itself, is a self-help network, with an extensive mutual-aid system characteristic of a membership organization."[2,p.216]

Twenty-five organizations (58%) responded to the questionnaire. Twenty sets of responses were returned by mail and the remaining five were recorded on follow-up phone calls.

The responding organizations were defined as follows:

Management sponsored EAPs	14
Hospitals (including one consortium)	3
Unions	7
City Agency	1
Total	25

The programs had been functional from under one year to thirty-five years. The number of employees served by each program ranged from three hundred to 185,000. The number of staff per program ranged from one to twenty. The number of staff does not appear to relate to the size of the organization. Union programs have the largest number of staff per program, averaging 9.2, while hospitals averaged 2.7 and management sponsored programs averaged 2.5. Eight programs had only one staff member. No correlation was found between the staff size and the utilization of groups.

Of the twenty-five respondents, twenty programs used groups, and five did not. In programs with one staff member, a 75% rate of group utilization was found.

GROUP USAGE BY ORGANIZATIONAL TYPE

Program Type	# used groups	# did not use groups
Management Sponsored	10	4
Union	6	1
Hospital	3	
City Agency	1	—
Total	20	5

The twenty organizations cited over eighty separate concerns, some specific, some general, that were addressed in groups. The following table organizes the concerns into these basic categories: I. Health, II. Mental Health, A. Individual, B. Family, III. Work Related Issues, IV. Concrete Issues and V. Miscellaneous.

Specific Concerns Addressed in Groups

(Where more than one organization cited the same issue, the number appears to the right of the issue in parenthesis.)

I. Health

   Alcoholism, recovering alcoholic or alcoholism in family (9)
   Breast Examination
   Cardiovascular Evaluation
   Cholesterol
   Choosing a physician
   Cigarette addiction
   Drugs (3)
   Fitness/choosing an exercise program
   Health care/coping with medical institutions (2)
   Hypertension
   Nutrition
   Weight Management (2)

II. Mental Health
    A. Individual   B. Family

Assertiveness
Coping with change
Depression
Death and Dying/
  Loss and grief
Personal Growth
Retirement,
  adjustment to
Stress (8)
Victim's assistance

Care of aging relative (3)
Domestic violence
Family problems
Parenting (3)
Selecting Daycare
Children and drugs
Understanding
  adolescence (2)
Single parents (4)
Work and family life

III. Work related issues
Newly hired employees
Job

problems
burnout
training

Management training (including use of the EAP) (7)
Problems of particular work units
Time management
Retirement planning (3)

IV. Concrete issues

Consumer affairs
Financial assistance
Housing

V. Miscellaneous

Mutual problems
Various issues

The respondents described the purpose of the groups as follows, choosing more than one answer, where applicable):

Purpose	# of organizations
To inform and educate	15
For mutual support	14

To enhance job functioning	6
Self help	1
Other	1

These answers emphasize helping individuals through group use over helping the organization directly (with the goal of producing better workers). However, several organizations specifically indicated that they do not do "therapy" groups.

Program design could be an important factor in determining utilization of the group format. Unfortunately, an important question was inadvertantly omitted from the questionnaire: a question that would have yielded information about whether the EAP provides information, assessment and referral only or whether it offers counseling and other social services, in addition. The former type of program is less likely to use groups. Future study is required to verify this conclusion which is based on information proferred but not requested from two of the programs which did not use groups: they said they did not themselves) provide services.

Next, group frequency was explored:

Frequency of meetings	# of organizations
Single sessions	10
Two to six sessions	8
Varied groups/Varied frequency	6
Ongoing	6
Other (annual, monthly, semi weekly)	3

Ongoing groups were found most frequently in union programs (four of the six) and least frequently in management sponsored programs. However, some ongoing groups could have been lost in the answer, "varied groups with varied frequency."

A wide range of professionals were represented in the role of group leader.

Leader	# of organizations
Mental health professional	13
Health care practitioner	7

Human resource personnel	2
Self help/employee led	4
Teacher/trainer/instructor	1
Student	4
Other (Lawyer, Senior Manager)	2

Students lead groups in unions and hospitals, but not in the fourteen management sponsored programs.

EAP programs evaluated their groups as follows: fourteen said they were very helpful, one said the evaluation was in progress and five did not respond to this question. Fourteen programs planned to expand group use, one did not, and one said that expansion depended on results of an evaluation which was in progress, and four did not answer that question. Reasons for expansion included, "groups are an effective modality" and a "cost effective program tool." The organizations that did not use groups gave these reasons: Not appropriate in setting (3), employees wouldn't participate (1), and no appropriate leader (1). The only union program that did not use groups was a job-match program for unemployed workers and even in this program, group use was projected for future use.

Two programs requested more information about how groups were used in other organizations. Three organizations who already used groups also requested such information, even though survey instructions aimed this question only at organizations which did not use groups. This may indicate a lack of information among EAP practitioners about current practices, policies and program designs in the field. While an exchange of information is clearly necessary, some organizations are reluctant (as was one bank which chose not to participate in the study), to share information about their program. That their employees have problems and that the organization responds to such problems is considered sensitive and private in some corporate cultures. Despite the growth in numbers of EAPs nationwide, some organizations still perceive that establishing an EAP in order to help the troubled worker as an intrusion into his/her private life. However, it may be possible that a group experience providing information and support may be viewed as less intrusive and could pave the way for introducing other needed social services.

The author expected that one of the uses of groups that would be identified in the study would be quality circles. However, this was not the case. When quality circles are utilized, they are sponsored not by the EAP but by either the Employee Relations Department or the Human Resources or Training Department of a corporation. Because the concept of quality circles may be of interest to social workers who in fact do lead some), this paper now offers a brief discussion of this method. "Since the late 1970's, . . . circles have been introduced at hundreds of American companies."[17,p.35] Quality circles involve group members in a decision making process about job related problems. Though more common in corporations, quality circles have begun to appear in the not-for-profit sector as well. In Michigan's Bay de Noc Community College, ". . . employees meet voluntarily every week to study on-the-job problems. Administrators agree to consider their recommended solutions and, in many cases, will adopt them."[18] At the Champion International Corporation in Connecticut, quality circle members have made changes in the chairs utilized by video-display operators, the decor of the office and, more significantly, in selling the concept of flextime to management.[17,p.34-6]

Because the study was designed to reflect some hands-on information about quality circles, one questionnaire was sent to a social work practitioner who had written about the use of quality circles in an advertising agency. One hundred and forty employees are served by this four year program with three staff members. The concerns addressed by the groups are: work related problems, research/technical skills and managerial skills. These groups function as either quality circles or training groups. The participants are research staff, clerical staff or sales staff. Group membership is related to job title. The purpose of these groups is to inform and educate, to enhance mutual support and improve job functioning. The groups have been evaluated as very helpful by the participants. Increased use of groups is planned because, "groups are a very effective medium for solving problems and training. People learn and are stimulated by the experience of others."[14] The group leader is either a mental health practitioner or human resource personnel.

CONCLUSIONS OF THE STUDY

Clearly the use of groups in industry has progressed from a "potential" or an "opportunity" to a reality. Although the study's findings are not necessarily transferable to other geographical areas or to all other EAPs, the reasons for group use and the types of issues addressed seem to parellel the underlying rationales for the development of EAPs: that an employee's personal/family life is not discrete from work life. In addition, the positive evaluations of group use plainly indicate a commitment to continued and expanded use of this modality.

The use of groups allows an EAP to reach far more employees than could be reached in individual counseling. Moreover, group participation is voluntary. It is a non-stigmatizing form of help, since a group experience can be utilized to gather information or to learn how others cope with similar situations, not because the employee is dysfunctional. In fact, groups can have special appeal to the high functioning but distressed individual, a population often not served in traditional mental health settings.

Expanded use of groups could indicate that social services at the worksite are being provided in a more benign and preventative atmosphere, a move away from the earlier model of mandatory supervisory referral for a troubled employee. The trend toward self-referral appears to be overtaking mandatory supervisory referrals as the primary route to the EAP as word spreads among employees of the assistance they have received. Participation in a group or workshop can be just the introductory experience that enables the worker to utilize counseling or other EAP services.

Conclusion

Additional study on group utilization in the industrial sector is clearly necessary. Equally important is the development of formalized information exchange programs for practitioners.

Groups are being utilized at the worksite in various ways that respond to diverse employee needs relating to their lives at work and at home. The benefits of group use in more traditional settings are transferable to the worksite. An understanding of the organizational culture, employee needs and specialized factors in worksite groups is crucial in the planning of groups. Solid planning and research will lead to broad acceptance and utilization of groups at the worksite. The dual concerns of industry for cost effective programs and improved employee health and productivity can make groups a very attractive complement to the individual mental health service delivery model.

REFERENCES

1. Hyman Weiner. "A Group Approach to Community Mental Health With Labor," *Social Work Practice*, 1967.
2. Paul Kurzman & Sheila Akabas. *Work, Workers and Work Organizations: A View From Social Work* (Englewood Cliffs, NJ: Prentice Hall, 1982).
3. "Social Work and the Workplace," Practice Digest, vol. 5, #2, September 1982, entire issue devoted to industrial social work.
4. "Employers Offering Seminars to Help the Working Parent," *New York Times*, June 23, 1983.
5. "Employers Offer Help in Divorces," *New York Times*, November 22, 1982.
6. E. Schein & W. Bennis. *Personal and Organizational Change Through Group Methods*, (New York: John Wiley and Sons, Inc. 1983).
7. L. Brown. "Mutual Help Staff Groups to Manage Work Stress," *Social Work With Groups*, vol. 7, #2, Summer 1984.
8. Sheila Akabas & Seth Akabas, "Social Services at the Workplace: New Resource for Management," *Management Review*, May 1982.
9. B. Feinstein & E. Brown. *The New Partnership: Human Services in Business and Industry* (Cambridge, MA: Schenkman, 1982).
10. Roxanne Mendelsohn. "The Emergence of Support Groups From an Employee Health Service," *Occupational Health Nursing*, May 1982.
11. Lawrence Shulman. *The Skills of Helping Individuals and Groups* (Itasca, IL: F.E. Peacock Publishers, 1984).
12. S. Wilson. *Confidentiality in Social Work: Issues and Principles* (New York: The Free Press, 1978).
13. M. Galinsky & J. Schopler. "Warning: Groups May Be Dangerous," Social Work, March 1977.

14. Nancy Petaja, M. S. W. Yankelovich, Skelly & White, quote from questionnaire.

15. M. Shain & J. Groenveld. *E.A.P.: Philosophy, Theory and Practice* (Lexington, MA: Lexington Books, 1980).

16. C. Winick. "A Labor Approach to Dealing With Alcohol Problems At the Workplace," Central Labor Council, 1982.

17. Naomi Barko. "Where Workers Speak and Bosses Listen," *Working Mother*, November 1985, pp. 34-36.

18. Liz McMillen. "College Employees Try 'Quality Circles' to Improve Administration, Curriculum," *The Chronicle of Higher Education*, Dec. 11, 1985.

19. Deanna L. Thompson. "Corporate Caring," *Piedmont Airlines*, January 1986.

20. Jeffrey Marvis. "The Psychological Route to Cutting Costs," *New York Times*, November 24, 1985.

Chinese Painting and Social Group Work

Annie Wu King

SUMMARY. Our pluristic society is ripe with many traditions upon which to draw. The concept of space in Chinese art may contribute to an enriched understanding of relationships within a group.

In your mind's eye look upon a Chinese painting of mountains, a winding river and perhaps a small boat in the distance, making its way up the watery path. There are mists and spaces, light and dark, all a part of the integrated whole.

Looking through journals on social work and group work, we find more and more articles on the use of social group work, peer support groups, self-help and mutual aid groups as will as networking in the natural support systems. Toseland and Hacker (1985) recently have suggested there are about one-half million self-help groups alone in this country. It appears that social group work is, and will be, of growing importance in the future.

In preparing for this future, I would like to suggest that as social group workers, we draw from the richer fabric of our worlds as a whole rather than restrict ourselves to the ingrown rituals of one tradition; that we allow ourselves the freedom to incorporate the paths, the mists and spaces of Chinese art, for example, in order to expand our understanding of our own smaller communities. This is not a new concept but lies, like a precious stone, in the folds of our social work family stories to be brought out, dusted off and shown to international guests in their visits to those settlement houses we think of so fondly. We are a nation of exciting racial ethnic diversification; unfortunately we sometimes forget this. I would therefore

Annie Wu King is a Practitioner and Graduate Student at the Center for Accessible Living, Louisville, Kentucky.

like to share with you my own personal perceptions as a woman and as an Amerasian.

My approach is basically structural, viewing the individual's problems as related to what is going on in society, in the family, or in the organization. This holistic approach is concerned not only with the parts but with the relationship of the whole, the "yin" and "yang" of the society, the relational intertwining of parts and a sensed balance within the universe. As social workers, we need to listen to the heartbeat of society, paying special attention to hurting populations in relation to the whole. I am reminded of the stories I was fascinated by as a teenager living in China. The ancient Chinese physician, when called in to diagnose a patient, especially a female patient, would sit respectfully beside the curtained bed, concentrating on the energy of the hurting part in relation to the whole as he felt the pulse of the patient. He would thus determine the disease and prescribe for it without having to examine in detail the particular painful area.

I am not suggesting that we shelter ourselves or those we work with behind curtains; I am suggesting that in these times of financial cutbacks, restricted services and thousands spent on research, we might do well to occasionally sit and listen to our collective heartbeat. It is as a woman I am learning to trust my sense of caring, inter-connectedness, and responsibility to the whole. As a woman I am learning not always to deny what I feel and what I perceive. It is as a woman that I sense deep loneliness in our society. As a woman, too, I am sure that paths in and out of the web of loneliness and alienation are never the same. The web itself may appear similar to others, yet is actually very different; the spaces and threads compose a unique whole.

Our attempts to escape from loneliness into relatedness has been researched and prescribed for in various ways. I remember an experience I had when I joined a T-group (sensitivity training group) after living in Central Java, Indonesia, for more than four years. During the mini-marathon at the close of the six weeks of regular meetings, I recall how surprised I was when someone told me that they had been upset with me because I was unwilling to share anything about myself. I realized then that I had absorbed more Javanese culture than I had been aware of. As I saw it, I had been quite open and willing to talk but was often "cut off" by others with their busy agenda to "get things out." To the American I was somehow lacking assertiveness and openness; to the Javanese I was behaving appropriately. The facilitator of the group acknowledged that I had made him uncomfortable because I was physically disabled and he, therefore, found it difficult to address me and especially to confront me! Systematized relating had not allowed for individual differences.

I came into conflict with values in this society which seem to be able to separate people into categories, cause and effect, group against group; perhaps this is the "yang" part of our society and results in a more psychomedical model. Perhaps it is our Protestant work ethic and rugged individualism that I, at times, take on uncomfortably. Hierarchical structures of power, right and wrong, earned justice, success to the "deserving" clash with my sense of interrelatedness and belonging, shared responsibility for the whole structure. As a social worker, what is my role in relation to those with whom I work? Must I be the giver and the taker? Do I need to have a sense of control in order to affect the change I desire? Am I sure of what change should be made? Am I able to enhance the self-esteem and growth of others as I, too, grow?

And so I come to attributes of my Asian self—a deep sense of extended relational network or community. Scenes from my life in both China and Indonesia pervade the underlying texture of my view of the society around me here. They mesh with the woman in me to suggest that the boundaries may not really be that distinct. There are scenes of grief and loss when family lines no longer divide people, when support and aid communicate caring. There are scenes of meetings with opposing factions where discussions are carried on calmly in order to "save face" for the losers. But are these scenes so unique to Asians? I have seen and heard some such expressions of community in Indiana and Kentucky. In groups of abused women, I have felt the sharing of strength and the caregiving that sustains a woman in crisis. And how many times I have heard the stories of relatedness during disasters or trouble. Yet so often in our organized work our basic belief in people seem to have eroded; we no longer trust others nor ourselves. We have let scientific research, technology and the politics of our advanced society distract from our view of the natural helping networks already existing, the potential for empowerment and healing that can withstand federal cutbacks and changes in government.

It is exciting to me that this particular mode of helping exists. As social workers we deal each day with the disenfranchized of our society — the isolated, the beaten, the castaways, people who are continually denied their humanity by mechanical institutional structures, by systems of noncommunication, by powerful hierarchical obstructions that prevent access to change and caring.

As a student, two contrasting group experiences stand out in my mind; both happen to be with abused women, but one was in a shelter for victims of spouse abuse while the other was in a mental health center. The women in the shelter guided the meeting, prodding, encouraging, crying with and advising each other. Almost all the members contributed to the discussion in their own way and as they left, they joked with each other and the staff worker. In the second experience, the therapists guided the conversation — questioning, pushing and cueing in other group members. When the meeting ended, the women left hurriedly while the therapists went in another direction.

I use this common example of one experience to highlight the fine line that seems to exist when we, as social group workers, attempt to provide the space in which people become connected, work on changing their own lives and their society, and gain a stronger sense of self-esteem without the authorization patterns of the past.

To me the excitement of social group work is the recognition that the so-called disenfranchized can give the very precious gifts of self-esteem and relatedness to each other. When control is not an issue for the group worker, participants have a better chance at empowerment. When the worker recognizes individuals as unique, community grows.

But is it not at this point we feel some uncertainty? How do we as social group workers deal with our need to achieve "success," to affect change? Do we dare trust the group members and the group process to accomplish what needs to be done? If I take a step back to allow another to step forward, will I lose my leadership position and end up following?

Chinese art is very special to me — it teaches much about life. My favorite is landscape painting. To fully appreciate the painting, one must step back and gaze on the painting as a whole. One's attention is engaged by the path or stream at the bottom of the painting which carries the viewer gently upwards and often into the distance, perhaps beside a miniature pavillion or between the mountain peaks. With the rising of the spirit comes a sense of wholeness. Although the details are important, the interrelatedness of the whole is the essence.

Blank space in Chinese painting is of great significance. Space is not just "that which is not filled" or "left over paper" — rather it is an integral part of the whole. Space can occur at the bottom, in the center, or upper part of the painting. It is of importance to an understanding of the painting.

I would suggest that in many of our groups we need to allow for the "flexibility of space" between the worker and the members. We can be an integral part of the scene without protruding into that space which allows the essence of the individual members to rise, to grow; space that respects the unique racial ethnic gifts of members as they shape the group and themselves. We speak of empowering others — what about space that allows others to empower themselves.

I remember a difficult lesson I had to learn when I first went to Java, Indonesia. Indonesian friends, teachers and students at the university where we taught would come to visit. Often they would stay a long time, sometimes sitting in silence. My western half of me experienced uneasiness. I tried to fill the space with questions. Gradually I began to understand and appreciate the silence, the space. Communication can continue in silence. They were not uncomfortable with silence — only I was until I could let go and enjoy the space, the other person and myself as a whole.

Those with whom we work probably have not had the luxury of giving; can we allow this to occur in our groups? How often have they been able to influence the direction of events? What growth can occur when members begin to take charge of the group — and their lives. We, as workers, in turn, can feel the security of space — a related, significant element of the whole — without which the painting would not be complete.

Perhaps we can borrow from Milton Erickson, trusting that within the individual lie resources upon to draw in finding answers. Space allows for that dawning of understanding and strength. Space gives support while remaining adaptable. Group experiences where members are in control or feel able to contribute to the progress of the meeting and each other expand the internal map of individuals upon which they can draw when needed. It can also expose them to the experiences of others and create new resources.

Allowing for space in a group is not always just the problem of a group worker or facilitator. Often group members themselves panic when the "worker" is not in control. During one session of the weekly peer-support group in an independent living center where people with various disabilities come together, the staff person, who strongly believes in the abilities of the group and the various individuals, sensed that some members had been turning too much to her for direction. She, therefore, announced to the group that she was no longer "mother." The reaction was immediate; one person wheeled his chair right out the door in a rage, another turned her chair around and stared out the window, while a third retreated into herself and did not speak again. Others ignored the worker's statement completely. During subsequent sessions, the peer-supporters were able to assume leadership roles and accept the staff member in a different space.

Space, perhaps, is a model we can learn to incorporate in our vision of the future even though we are not comfortable with it at present. It is a concept that can contribute to growth and fullness, a concept that allows for the rich variety of people that make up our communities.

As a path in a Chinese painting, I have wandered from one place to the next, disappearing in spaces of emptiness to reappear in another direction. My vision for the future of social group work is one of textured designs woven together in a fabric of rich international traditions — open to the varied lives of those we serve yet creating the possibility of relatedness with spaces where people may grow into fuller human beings.

REFERENCE

Toseland, R. W. & Hacker, L. (1985). Social workers' use of self-help groups as a resource for clients, in *Social Work*, 30, No. 3 (May-June), pp. 232-237.

The Use of the Group
in Assisting Graduate Students
to Cope with a Systems Crisis:
Labor Disruption/Strike
in Field Placement

Muriel Gladstein

SUMMARY. A discussion of the use of the mutual aid group to facilitate students' coping with systems' crises, in both the academic and field placement environments. Illustrations highlight the opportunities, provided by the group, for students' enhanced development of their professional selves from events, originally experienced as crises.

INTRODUCTION

This paper will describe the use of the group, for mutual aid and professional growth, in coping with crises brought about by strikes

Muriel Gladstein is an assistant professor at Hunter College School of Social Work, City University of New York.

or potential strikes in the field work placement of students. The two examples to be detailed are a work stoppage, and a strike.

Background

All students at the Hunter College School of Social Work have experience with formal participation in school designed groups. Their participation in these groups helped to provide the experiences and foundation needed for their positive use of the group developed to deal with the resolution of crisis arising from situations in their agency placements.

Almost all applicants to the Hunter College School of Social Work are interviewed in "group admissions interviews." Once admitted as students in the program, they meet on a regular basis with the faculty member who is assigned as their advisor. This is discussed more freely in a later section.

The Group Admissions Process

At the Hunter College School of Social Work, group admissions interviews are scheduled with most applicants to the program. Initially, it was assumed that seeing applicant in a group could be illuminating. However, the use of the group rather than the individual interview is also seen to be a more economical use of scarce faculty time. (In certain, few, special situations, applicants are still seen individually.)

The group interview has been conceptualized as being useful for both the admissions committee faculty and for the applicants. The applicants learn about the organization of the school, the mission of the school, and the choices they have in relation to their education. More questions are raised by six or eight students together with one faculty member than any one student thinks of or dares to raise in an individual interview! Applicants have the opportunity to experience other applicants, a faculty representative, and the physical environment of the school. They are also able to observe their own behavior in a somewhat anxiety producing situation.

Faculty has the opportunity to share information; to observe an applicant's capacity for inter-group relationship, for mutual aid to other group members, for monitoring their individual anxiety, for sharing or withholding content that is appropriate or inappropriate in a group admissions interview. Informal data suggests that the success rate in determining via the group interview, which applicants are suitable for entry to the program has been equal to the merits of our judgments based on individual interviews.

THE FACULTY ADVISEMENT PROCESS

A second institutionalized use of the group has been in fulfilling the function of faculty advising. The faculty advisor serves as group leader; the advisees are members of the group. The function of the advisor is to assist and evaluate student progress in all areas of the educational experience; to accomplish this, close collaboration with the agency field instructor(s) is necessary. The roles carried by the faculty advisor include: orientation, teaching, consultation, evaluation and accreditation, administration and at times, advocacy. One rationale for the use of the group in the faculty advising process was that it was thought to be a good use of faculty time. It was also assumed that there would be many positive outcomes.

Faculty advisors and the students for whom they have the advisement responsibility are a "natural" group, which has both task and growth objectives. To paraphrase Gitterman,

> By its very nature, the group mutual aid system universalizes peoples' problems, reducing isolation and stigma. The group has inherent potential for a multiplicity of helping relationships. Collective strength and power is developed as is the force in helping people to act and gain greater control and mastery over their environments.[1]

Mary Louise Somers, in a paper entitled "The Small Group in Learning and Teaching" writes about the cohesive small groups providing effective support for the learner in his/her encounters with the anxiety producing aspects of learning. The group, if strong, can also encourage the expression of differences. The faculty member who trusts the learning group develops a new kind of knowledge and understanding, and frequently a kind of insight and self-knowledge which is an invaluable part of a teacher's professional self.[2]

Faculty also has an opportunity to model group interaction skills; to validate students' contributions; to experience students' peer interaction and learning; and to demonstrate and underline the process of continuing professional development. The opportunities for rehearsal and role playing are increased with the larger cast of "actors."

For students who are not enrolled in group work courses and are not practicing group work, the group faculty advising process provides the opportunity for experiencing the power and the process of the group.

Kadushin's material in relation to group supervision is also germane to group faculty advising. He mentions the opportunities: for lateral or peer to peer teaching, for the display of emotional support, sympathy, and praise. The feeling of belonging is reinforced by experiences which are gratifying and morale building.[3] In group faculty advising, as in all teaching of social work students, it is essential that the focus be educational not therapeutic; this needs to be made explicit in the contract with the group.

The faculty member must also attempt to:

1. Diminish feelings of "sibling" rivalry and competition among members and
2. Encourage and support students felt and demonstrated experiences in stimulating and focusing group interaction.

The Use of Mutual Aid Groups in: Helping Students Cope with Systems Crises

Schwartz's criteria for the mutual aid groups is applicable and needs only to substitute the word "faculty member" for the word "worker" and the word "student" for "client." To quote,

> A mutual aid group is a helping system in which students need each other as well as the faculty member. This need to use each other, to create not one but many helping relationships, is a vital ingredient of the group process constitutes a common

need over and above the specific tasks for which the group was formed.[4]

The principles and concepts to be discussed in the two detailed examples would be applicable to the use of the mutual aid group in other crisis situations as well, i.e.,

1. The need to confront feelings around the termination of a student or a faculty member.
2. The need to deal with the feelings and consequences, in an agency, of the curtailment of services because of termination of funding.
3. The need to deal with the feelings and required interventions caused by an epidemic on a medical service, in a hospital placement.

Work Stoppage and Strike: The Threat of the Premature Termination of Field Work

The two detailed examples of the use of mutual aid groups to help students deal with crises in systems have important commonalities; they both threatened the students' opportunities to continue with the field placement part of their education, and they both necessitated thinking and discussing conflictual value and ethical issues.

An unplanned departure from the field not only would prevent students from serving their clients, from continuing to apply learned principles to practice, but would also separate the student from the mentor whom Berengarten describes as the field instructor who is "closest to the student in action, in feeling, in thinking, and in behaving."[5]

Both crises occurred as a result of the consequences of the unionization of professional social workers. The opportunity to deal with some of the values of the profession was appreciated by school and, in the first instance, by field faculty. Dr. Harold Lewis's discussion of the critical aspect of values and ethics in the development of skill supported the work being done in the groups.[6] It was integral, not superfluous, to the students' professional development. The work done in the first example occurred in the agency; the second group met at school.

First Example

In the first instance, the agency setting was a bi-agency placement: a hospital and a community center. The two field instructors of the student unit met with the entire student unit once a month to discuss "professional issues," this complemented students weekly individual field instruction. With the threat of a work stoppage in the hospital, the unionization of professionals became the issue. Meetings were scheduled on a once a week basis and continued, at the community center, when the strike became a reality. The field instructors needed to prepare for helping the students to confront and deal with difficult professional realities and met first together and then together with agency administrators and school faculty.

Educational field assignments were a minimal problem as only one of the two agencies was threatened with a strike. The students' assignments in the community center were expanded.

Some of the professional issues dealt with were:

> The position of our professional organization; the National Association of Social Workers whose policy position states: "social workers should be guided by 'professional values' when they participate in collective bargaining."

> The professional value which supports the rights of individuals to attempt to enhance their living conditions, even if a strike meant that workers' services to clients would be temporarily interrupted and delivered by administrative staff.

> The students were actors in a scenario written by other professionals.

Consequences

> Students experienced clients as "whole people," not only as patients with illnesses requiring hospitalization, as they discussed with them the realities of what staff was experiencing in the process of negotiation. Clients shared with the students their own experience as workers and as union members.

The students saw the patient experiencing, during the strike, an entire system that cared and continued serving them, expanding the patient-worker relationships for the patient.

For the student, this meant that they also saw themselves giving service, but as a part of the service delivery system.

Most important was students experiencing the critical importance of institutions and institutional supports for patients and staff. The students witnessed the compatibility of unionization with being a professional. They felt positive about realizing that they, in the future, as workers would be capable of advocating for themselves.

Last, but hardly least, students and patients lived through a "mini-termination" experience which helped to prepare for the end of semester termination.

Second Example

An agency strike at the end of a spring semester of a two-year graduate program promoted the formation of a mutual aid group which significantly enhanced the professional development of the involved students. At that time a major consortium of hospitals including medical and psychiatric facilities was confronted by a strike of staff members. Social workers were members of the same union as the striking workers and supported the strike by absenting themselves from work for the three-week period. This medical consortium has a strong commitment to patient care and also to the education of professionals of many disciplines.

Our school of social work is structurally organized into five concentrations based on the identification of human needs and the resources required to meet these needs. The six first and second year students involved had been, because of this organizational plan, in classes together during their first year of school; the faculty advisor-liaison person to the consortium taught in the health concentration. Finally, the agencies, also members of health concentration, collaborated in an advisory capacity, with campus faculty in relation to curriculum. (The curriculum organization summarized here is spelled out in greater detail by Caroff and Mailick, 1980.)[7] Therefore, a tightly knit group of field people, students and faculty were the persons concerned with the strike situation.

Stated school policy mandates that students should not enter an agency in which there is a strike for several reasons: 1. normal educational opportunities would be impossible; 2. students might be put into a situation of "scabbing"; 3. physical safety might be in jeopardy. The policy reads as follows:

> If an agency to which students have been assigned has a period when services are disrupted due to a breakdown in labor-management relationships, strikes, etc., it is expected that the school will be so informed of these developments by the agency executives so that the effect and implications for the student program in the field can be assessed and suitable plans made for the students' ongoing training.

> If such difficulties occur, the School takes the position that if the atmosphere of the agency is no longer conducive to an educationally sound training program, due to the strained and disruptive personnel situation, disruption in program services, and unavailability of field instructor staff, the students should be withdrawn from that field experience. Based on a careful review, a decision is made by the School. In such instances, the students will be withdrawn from the agency. The students, however, will be expected to maintain their professional responsibility to clients, advising them of their absence and informing and planning with them about the appropriate channels available for any emergency services. Students are expected to bring all their dictation up to date so records can be available in case action needs to be taken.

> The School in these instances takes responsibility for planning and arranging *substitute field work activities for students* either at the School, or in other centers.[8]

This policy does not permit students placed in agencies where social workers are on strike to make their own decision about continuing or not continuing in field work (during a strike situation).

The principles governing the school's response to this particular strike situation were based on the assumption that the situation would be temporary, and, in fact, presented an impromptu opportunity to deal experientially with professional issues and practices. It was also anticipated that alternate learning opportunities could be planned.

In consultation with the field work department, administration, the faculty advisor, who had the responsibility of the liaison function between students and agency, and students, it was decided that the students would not be transferred to other placements. This would have been difficult to do. It was also felt that they would, hopefully, eventually have the opportunity to continue with their clients and their field instructors and to end planfully and professionally. This was the eventual outcome. The structure and learning opportunities designed were described after a discussion of the nature of the group.

The agencies supported the School's decision and, in fact, seemed relieved at not needing to have to deal with the issues of student education at this time.

As in the previously described strike situation, students had genuine concern about their clients. The second year students were also concerned that an interruption of field work would interfere with their graduation and with their ability to find employment after graduation. The first year students, a smaller and less cohesive group, were at a different point in their learning. They found being away from the agency a relief, initially, from the required psychological and physical demands. The entire group experienced some of this relief. There were concomitant guilt feelings that some of their focus was more on themselves than on their clients. Their honesty and openness in risking and sharing these feelings, felt to be "taboo," was a major positive in developing self-awareness during the shared experience of "being on strike." A second major positive was the cohesiveness experienced by the group which had strong feelings of identification with each other, the agency, staff and faculty. The students also experienced the educational institution to be very supportive of their unique experience. The organizational structure of concentrations was a most positive force in the outcome of the experience for students and faculty.

The decision that students not be replaced in different agencies for the remainder of the semester (about six weeks) necessitated formulation of additional policy which provided structure and boundaries for the students. It was decided that:

1. Second year students' graduation would not be jeopardized.
2. First year students would move to second year on schedule.
3. Alternate learning opportunities would be provided by the School.
4. Students would also be encouraged to pursue individual professional interests.
5. The faculty advisor would be available to coordinate additional learning opportunities.
6. Students would be helped to develop accountability structures; i.e., logs and reports. This was seen as essential as it was necessary that standards of graduation be fulfilled.
7. Regular and frequent meetings of the group led by the advisor, was to be the process in which these policies were to be operationalized.

In fact, these meetings were the core that helped this experience be successful. The meetings maintained group support, provided for the exchange of a wide range of information including information about the strike and about planned activities. It was never less than an excellent example of the group as a "mutual aid system" (Shulman, 1979).[9]

Among the issues dealt with was the conflict created for social workers when there was disagreement between the objectives of the systems and the roles with which they were learning to be affiliated. As social workers they felt both an obligation to their clients and an obligation to staff who were on strike. They had no input in decisions. Their actions were decided for them. While the students did not necessarily resolve these conflicts, the discussions heightened their awareness of the issues involved. They felt comforted by mutual support and by "being in the same boat" with each other.

Finally, for the group of students, the opportunity was presented to experience what many of their blue collar clients experienced in their work lives and in their roles as union members. Though the students missed only three weeks of field work, they were away a fourth week as it was Spring recess. Their field instructors had the opportunity, in this week, to work through some of their own feelings about the strike and to prepare for the return of the students.

The fact that coverage for clients was arranged for by agency administration and staff was a source of professional pride and comfort to students, staff and faculty.

Epstein, in "Professional Orientation and Conflict Strategies" (1970) explores the social action effects of the role orientations of social workers. He found that a bureaucratic orientation is found to be conservatizing, a client orientation radicalizing and a profession orientation, when taken alone is neither.[10]

The students involved in the strike situation felt that their support of the union (not individually arrived at decisions) was radicalizing for them as individuals. In the long run, the decision was oriented to clients who would be served by appropriately paid, valued, social workers who had the strength and power to advocate for what they felt were their entitlements. The students certainly had more of a "client" than a "bureaucratic" orientation, they had found a "strength in numbers."

Some of the activities engaged in by group members, during the strike, included visits to other agencies which broadened their knowledge of services being offered, clients being served and treatment modalities being used. Lectures, presentations, and films while scheduled for other purposes in some instances, were also utilized as alternate field work learning opportunities. The group shared responsibility for a resume writing session and heard one group member discuss a political situation which was of mutual concern. Some students, taking on individual responsibilities for problem solving, arranged to return to spend more time at agencies, with input from the faculty advisor, where they had worked prior to coming to school. In one instance, a student was still employed on a part-time basis and arranged for more work hours in that agency. All students reported, at the end of the strike, that there had not been one field day in which they had not had a "social work related" experience. The educational coordinator at the striking institution also helped to arrange some time for the students in programs where the institutions were not on strike.

This continuing connection to the social work profession, the strong support of faculty and of agencies connected to the school was crucial to the high morale, the developing professionalism, and the fulfillment of educational requirements. Students found themselves connected to the entire educational (school-agency) system and not to individual faculty and to individual agencies. To quote from one student's log: "I was surprised at the number of faculty who knew the striking student and expressed interest, concern, and support." It was critical learning time, this "end phase" described by Robinson (1978) as the phase of learning in which the student prepares to leave the situation and to take over what she/he has learned as his own.[11]

In spite of all the learning opportunities, there were some difficulties in the existing situation dealing with the ambivalence in relationships with students not on strike who were resentful of the striking students' "free time." This time was being used for new and exciting learning experiences and for some work on academic requirements. The group of students eventually talked essentially with each other and with interested and concerned faculty. This helped them to cope with their increasing anxieties.

As the strike continued, with little optimism and varied reports about the status of negotiations, some of the expressed feelings were: "What if the strike does not end before the end of the semester?" "Who will write my final evaluation?" "Will I get a chance to terminate with my clients?" "In class and everywhere else everyone is discussing termination," and "I feel in limbo." Some quotes from written comments submitted document some of what has been discussed, especially the fact that much growth in self-awareness and professionalism occurred during this experience.

A second year student wrote: "The strike made me aware of professional issues which I may face again. It was advantageous to be in a situation where I had help in working them through."

Another second year student wrote: "I never realized the importance of work. It gives one purpose, direction, motivation, and boundaries. It gives one the freedom to engage in other activities."

Equal care was given to the process of the students' return to the agency at the end of the strike. The students found that they did not have to "begin all over again." Their clients had received necessary services, were reasonably understanding of the situation, and not angry at them. A positive was the opportunity to "compare notes" with the students from other schools, with whom they had had little contact during the strike. The final evaluations written by the field instructors had little if any reference to the impact of the strike as an interruption or deterrent in the learning experience. The (value) issues worked on, in group, were numerous: 1. "the right to self-determination" is not a universal given; 2. the students' behavior was proscribed by the school; 3. conflict may exist between roles; the role of "worker" may require some change in the role of "deliverer of service"; 4. the reality that clients are connected to systems and not to individual faculty and to individual agencies. Finally, the students experienced the new strength that developed from "living through" uncertainty along with the positive feelings resulting from some resolution of conflict experienced by them and by agency staff.

The students' logs, a recording of their daily activities and impressions of these activities, provided documentation that: their time was being spent on professional activities; detailed the new learning that was taking place; provided content for sharing between students and with the faculty member.

The faculty person kept not a log, but a schedule of the students' daily activities which provided for the students a sense of structure and also an accountability measure to them and to the educational system.

Implication for Educators

Some "helpful hints" to other professional educators engaged in a similar situation, interruption of field work because of a work stoppage or strike situation in an agency include the following suggestions. A school can help to make this potential crisis a positive experience by 1. assuming responsibility for certain educational decisions; i.e., field attendance or nonattendance; field replacement or non-replacement; 2. the development of alternative educational programs, if students are not in the field; 3. the use of the group as a "mutual aid" support group, if more than one student is involved.

The length of the strike; the time it occurs in the academic year; the cohesiveness of the students and faculty; the resources of the school (academic and field) were all crucial variables in the outcome of the experience described and of other such experiences.

Social work educators need to address their own feelings in relation to union activities in the profession if they are to help students to confront the tension of the unknown experiences of all learning situations, particularly those experiences presenting conflict.

If we as professionals are to help our students to deal with the multiple issues raised by a labor situation, we need to be aware of our feelings, experiences, biases and conflicts; assume the responsibility of educators for the profession; and finally, be creative in the development of learning opportunities.

The students involved in the situation described their understanding of the compatibility of unions in professionalism. Many expressed similar sentiments too, "I feel at an advantage to have been able to experience this situation and to have worked it through in the way that I did. The strike was a situation which solidified the involved students with each other and with the school."

They understood, as expressed by Weissman, Epstein and Savage (1983) that unions can be an effective force for increasing wages and job security; for allowing workers to feel more independence; for permitting workers to negotiate with less fear of reprisal.[12]

Not all learning in professional school is technical; the learning acquired in a social sense in this experience helped to develop some commitment to particular ideas regarding the purposes and the practice of the profession.

CONCLUSION

Planning and preparation in developing groups for students in crises are critical activities. Educational institutions need to use their resources, to demonstrate and model what they teach about the importance and usefulness of the group process by providing students, when appropriate, with life experiences.

The role of a faculty member as leader and the students as participants in mutual aid groups dealings with educational crises has been described.

Finally, in this era of the commemoration of the life and work of Bertha Capen Reynolds,

In the history of unionization in social work, it is impossible to separate the two motives of protesting one's own condition as a worker and safeguarding the right to treat clients ethically.[13]

REFERENCES

1. Alex Gitterman. "The Development of Group Services, Social Work With Groups in Maternal and Child Health." *Conference Proceedings June 1979*. Columbia University School of Social Work and Roosevelt Hospital Department of Social Work.

2. Mary Louise Somers "The Small Group in Learning and Teaching." Council on Social Work Education.

3. Alfred Kadushin (1976). *Supervision in Social Work*. Columbia University Press, New York and London.

4. William Schwartz (1961). "The Social Worker in the Group" in *New Perspectives in Services to Groups*" (New York: National Association of Social Workers), p. 18.

5. Sidney Berengarten (1961). "Educational Issues in Field Instruction in Social Work." *Social Service Review,* Vol. XXXV, No. 3, September.

6. Harold Lewis (1982). *The Intellectual Base of Social Work Practice,* The Lois and Samuel Silberman Fund, New York, The Haworth Press.

7. Phyllis Caroff and Mildred Mailick (1980). *Social Work In Health Services*, New York, Prodist.

8. Hunter College School of Social Work, City University of New York, *Field Work Manual*, 1984.

9. Lawrence Shulman (1979). *The Skills of Helping*. F.E. Peacock Publishers, University of British Columbia. (The dynamics of the mutual aid process as spelled out by Shulman include: sharing of data, a dialectical process [the discussion of ideas, the modification of ideas, and the introduction of new ideas], the discussion of "taboo" areas, listening to each other with individuals discovering that they owned emotions of which they were unaware, the experiencing of the reality that all members were in the "same boat," making feelings less threatening and easier to deal with, emerging mutual support [empathic feelings were given and received] mutual demand, individual problem solving, rehearsing, and, finally, the experience of finding strength in numbers).

10. Irwin Epstein (1978). "Professional Role Orientations and Conflict Strategies," AMS Press, Inc.

11. Virginia Robinson (1983). *The Development of a Professional Self: Teaching and Learning in Professional Helping Services*, Philadelphia, Temple University Press.

12. Harold Weissman, Irwin Epstein, and Andrea Savage (1983). *Agency-Based Social Work: Neglected Aspects of Clinical Practice*, Philadelphia, Temple University Press.

13. Bertha Capen Reynolds. *Report for the United Seaman's Service* undated.

Changing the Silence: Communicating About the Nuclear Threat

Betty Levin

SUMMARY. Most people are numbed about the nuclear danger. At the Symposium nuclear workshop, participants transformed their numbing to action. The social group work profession is challenged to face the nuclear threat and brings its unique skills and cherished tradition of social action to this work as a "call to life."

The nuclear threat is a subject most people would rather avoid, a condition described as "psychic numbing" by psychiatrist Robert Lifton. Yet a modern-day Pandora's box has produced nuclear armaments that individuals and society cannot continue to ignore. "Changing the Silence," the workshop presented at the Seventh Annual Symposium on the Advancement of Social Work with Groups, encourages participants to express their feelings about living with the nuclear threat. The goal is changing their silence and numbing to awareness and response. Numbing represents an expression of powerlessness whereas awareness opens the possibility for empowerment and action.

The denial, suppression, and repression in numbing are ego-dystonic behaviors. They rob the individual of self-knowledge that can contribute to a more satisfying life. Much of mental health work with clients is to help them counter their denial defenses. The denial of the nuclear threat is a higher order of seriousness, and according

Betty Levin, Clinical Practice and Clinical Supervisor, Millburn, New Jersey.

to Goldman and Greenberg of the Psychiatry Task Force, Physicians for Social Responsibility (1982), represents the ultimate mental health problem. They state, "It is time for the mental health profession to treat the escalating nuclear arms race as our society's most urgent mental health problem, or we may never have the opportunity to treat any other problem" (p. 581). They exhort mental health professionals, as "agents of change," to become involved. Richard Barnet (1982), Senior Fellow, Institute of Policy Studies, discussing fantasy and realities of the arms race, concludes, "The primary mental health task in this country is to liberate the energies and the feelings of empowerment in our citizens so that we can address this task even as we fight to move the shadow of nuclear destruction from our lives" (p. 589).

The model for the "Changing the Silence" workshop is termed "despair and empowerment." It is a group-experienced process based on the concepts developed by Joanna Macy (1983), Chellis Glendinning (1984, 1987) and others on how the numbing of fear and helplessness can be relinquished and transformed into personal power. Others advocate similar group experiences to achieve empowerment. Harris Peck (1984), Professor Emeritus, Department of Psychiatry, Albert Einstein College of Medicine, discusses a group approach which "enables participants to claim the competence, power, and creativity they have manifested in other life areas and bring it (sic) to bear on the problems posed by the nuclear danger" (p. 226). Charles Garvin (1984) identifies empowerment as a need in coping with many social problems including threat of warfare: "The challenge to group work is to strengthen or create ways of working with groups that are responsive to these issues. One of the crucial ways is to help group members overcome feelings of powerlessness and futility . . ." (p. 18).

The process of these despair/empowerment workshops involves three components. Participants are helped to 1. relinquish the numbing and allow force of feelings to emerge; 2. express freely whatever feelings are there—sad, angry, helpless (called "despairwork"): and 3. discover a sense of power and competency that can be channeled into constructive response (called "empowerment").

PSYCHIC NUMBING

The first component of these workshops, helping people overcome psychic numbing, represents a major hurdle. Even those individuals who actively seek to attend are usually shut down about their feelings.

This phenomenon was first described by Lifton (1983) as characteristic of survivors of the atomic destruction in Hiroshima, ". . . the mind being severed from its own psychic forms" (p. 174). This keeps the fear and helplessness out of awareness. Even in less traumatic experiences, denied feelings are not available to the individual for appropriate response. In conditions of threat to safety and survival, this numbing becomes counterproductive. Individuals render themselves helpless to cope, immobilizing themselves in the face of danger. Their protective numbing is no protection at all in this "catch 22" syndrome.

For those participants in the workshop who can relinquish numbing, they must go to the next stage. As they become familiar with their deep feelings, they need opportunity to process the emerging despair.

DESPAIRWORK

Despairwork is based on five principles: 1. feelings of pain for our world are natural and healthy; 2. pain is morbid only if denied; 3. information alone is not enough; we need to process this information on the emotional level; 4. unblocking repressed feelings releases energy, clears the mind; 5. unblocking our pain for the world reconnects us with the larger web of life (Macy, 1983, pp. 22-23). Despair acknowledged, accepted and expressed as inner pain parallels the work of Kübler-Ross (1969) on death and dying. Glendinning (1987) characterizes the process as a "rite of passage" for mourning and transition. When shared in a supportive environment, new clarity, power and vision can emerge. Macy emphasizes that despairwork is consciousness-raising and can be deeply meaningful even short of empowerment: "Through our despair something more profound . . . comes to light. It is our interconnectedness . . . a sense of mutual belonging (to the planet) so real that the response is one of wonder, even joy" (1981, p. 47).

EMPOWERMENT

Denial of pain is often denial of power (McVeigh, 1984). Through despairwork, blocked energy becomes accessible to reclaim power and kindle vision for constructive action. Empowerment contributes to "compassion, community and commitment to act" (Macy, 1983, p. iii).

Julian Rappaport (1981) characterizes empowerment as a social change system and repudiation of paternalism. It insists on individuals participating in actions that affect their welfare. For a stunning example of empowerment of a disenfranchised population, see O'Sullivan, Waugh and Espeland (1984), "The Fort McDowell Yavapai, From Pawn to Powerbrokers."

Charles Kieffer (1984) declares empowerment is coming of age in the '80s, rooted in social action of the '60s and self-help movement of the '70s (p. 10). He states further, "The fundamental empowering transformation, then, is in the transition from sense of self as helpless victim to acceptance of self as assertive and efficacious citizen" (p. 32), all part of a long-term process of adult learning and development.

WORKSHOP DESCRIPTION AND PROCESS

The workshop is a 2-hour group process that includes a video/film and guided fantasies. The process starts with the film, "Changing the Silence" (Intersection Associates and Maya Gillingham, 1983), from which the workshop derives its title. Created by a group of high school students, the teenagers poignantly express despair that they may never grow up because of nuclear war and are angry that neither parents nor teachers will talk with them about their fears. After the film, the workshop participants divide into small groups for response and discussion. For most people, it is their first opportunity to speak about living with the nuclear threat. Some "change the silence," and psychic numbing starts to yield.

At almost every workshop, someone recalls childhood days at school, crouching under desks during atomic bomb drills. They express incredulity at the foolishness and naiveté of misguided officials who promoted such futile gestures. Their tone suggests feelings of betrayal and questioning of assumptions under which government leaders are presently functioning. Some comments are searing. One woman wonders, as she sends her young daughter to school, will a sudden nuclear attack prevent her from ever seeing her again? A couple, both successful professionals and devoted parents, tell of a family plan worked out with their adult children. If there is sufficient warning of a nuclear attack, they will all gather at their beloved country home to perish together. Many participants state they hope to be at ground zero when it happens. The use of the word "when" creeps into the dialogue. There is a tone of inevitability.

Some group members resist expressing feelings and resort to didactic material and debate. Others are unable to speak and remain in silence. In private afterwards, some have told the facilitator their fears were too painful to discuss openly. Whatever their participation, for almost all, the workshop serves as a consciousness-raising experience. For those people who discover new founts of energy and want to become involved, the follow-up brainstorming session (Formica, 1986) links those with common interests for possible action.

What qualities contribute to the despair/empowerment process? First, the teenagers in the film serve as *role models* for expression of anger and pain. This film presentation, combined with gentle questioning, i.e., "do you share some of the feelings expressed in the film?" serve as implicit *permission* to express what has been hidden. The *acceptance* and *non-judgmental* attitudes of the group establish a *safe* and *supportive environment* so that participants will not feel maudlin, "sick," or criticized for feeling as they do. As they start to reveal their sorrow and anguish, others join in their own expressions. Feelings become *validated* as participants recognize their own feelings in others. People discover *they are not alone* in their pain and helplessness. These *public acknowledgements* build momentum. The removal of denial, release of feelings unblocking of energy can lead to desire for action. Even without empowerment, there develops a feeling of commonality in a vast human problem.

SYMPOSIUM WORKSHOP

In the "Changing the Silence" workshop presented at the Symposium, the experience took on a totally unique form. Among the eight participants, almost all were social workers, most were socially-aware individuals and a few had been activists in the civil rights and Vietnam War eras. This altered the process and outcome significantly.

Immediately following the viewing of the film, the group shared feelings openly and quickly. Several people expressed frustration and disillusionment in trying to make impact on the arms race. They spoke bitterly of the futility of petitions, phone calls, tying ribbons around the Pentagon (a reference to the commemoration of the 40th anniversary of the bombing of Hiroshima). As expression and interaction increased, feelings became heightened. Frustration became charged with anger.

With the sharing of common concerns and passions, the group moved toward cohesiveness. The "burned-out" feelings were transformed to potent ones. Leadership emerged within the group, and suggestions were made for action. Some ideas were too complicated, time-consuming and impractical to be undertaken at that time. The problem-solving, reality-testing of decision making was in process. The group wanted immediate action. If there was any credibility in action, it should happen at this Symposium, at this hotel, now. No guided fantasies were needed: the group was immersed in the reality of the moment. The facilitator discarded the model in favor of the organic flow of a workshop that the participants themselves were shaping.

The group agreed on a plan of action. They would write a resolution to President Reagan and Secretary Gorbachev, as the two leaders were preparing for the Geneva summit meeting two weeks hence, asking for a cessation of nuclear arms proliferation. The group would try to bring the resolution to the conference itself. There was a conference luncheon scheduled in twenty minutes; could it be read there? As the group composed the resolution, they simultaneously discussed how to get permission to have it introduced at the luncheon. No one knew the chairperson at the luncheon, but someone knew someone who would be seated on the podium . . . perhaps it could be arranged. If that obstacle were overcome, then the group would also ask permission to circulate the White House Comment Desk phone number at the luncheon for attendees to telephone their personal messages to the President.

Permissions were obtained. The workshop had now moved into the larger convention. The resolution was read, the phone number circulated and another announcement made: the workshop would continue after the luncheon in the lobby of the hotel. Two new participants joined the group in the lobby. Afternoon plans were cancelled and the group, armed with the now-duplicated resolution, swept the lobby obtaining signatures. The effort continued into the next day. Eight members of the original workshop made impact on several hundred attendees at the larger conference, and an important message was sent to world leaders at a momentous time in history.

FROM EMPOWERMENT TO SOCIAL ACTION

The Symposium workshop was unique in that participants quickly felt empowered to take action. Occurring first in the workshop, the empowerment was transformed into social action within the Symposium community and eventually expressed at the international level. This was unusual not only for a two-hour workshop but that it occurred among individuals essentially strangers working under stringent time limits. The fervent response at the Symposium workshop exceeded any previous experience before or since.

What were the characteristics of the workshop that produced social action? As we examine models of group organization and social action, we can highlight which qualities and processes were present in the Symposium experience and which were absent. Perhaps this will suggest how models may be modified or amplified to produce more effective results and concomitantly, how the despair/empowerment workshops may be productively altered as well.

First, let us examine leadership roles in group organization and how they functioned in the Symposium workshop. Grosser (1979) distinguishes between the leadership styles of *enabler*, *broker*, *ad-*

vocate and *activist*. At the Symposium workshop, leaders started as *enablers*, clear about their own goals in helping participants reduce numbing and express feelings, but impartial as to how far participants would move in the process. The ultimate goal of empowerment was left to individuals to discover as they worked through the process. As participants worked cohesively to determine a collective action, the leaders shifted to a *broker* role. They asked clarifying questions when discussion became too diffuse and suggested actions became too impractical. When the group's plan of action was clearly defined, the leaders joined them as *advocates* and became partisans in the plan. Several participants became the new leaders as the group looked to them for direction even as they contributed their energy and ideas. The group was not fully in a social action mode. Social worker as *activist* is often seen as unprofessional and forfeiting the traditional neutral position. In the Symposium workshop, leaders were first neutral but allowed themselves to be incorporated into the process to join the activism.

Thus, it can be seen that varying leadership styles were utilized at the Symposium workshop, appropriate to the fast-moving process that was developing. This was a crucial aspect of the process. Yet it represents a departure from usual leadership roles that appear to remain constant in group organization. This suggests that activists could profitably explore flexibility in leadership roles. Also, within the enabler role, despairwork with client populations may well be included as part of the activists' armamentarium. Many clients' helplessness blocks constructive energy that could be working for their legitimate rights.

In Carniol's (1976) model of social action process, he explicates the following phases, 1. identification of injustice; 2. defining the position and seeking remedies; 3. building support; 4. mobilizing pressure; 5. sustaining reaction; 6. transforming values and structures.

The social action at the Symposium workshop paralleled Carniol's model in several respects but was most notable—and it's greatest weakness—where it departed. It was essentially a Carniol model in the first three processes: expressing anger over the arms race, pushing for immediate action and building and receiving support in the Symposium community. Hereafter, the social action process faltered seriously. Though dramatic, the workshop action was essentially a "one-shot" affair. The group never ventured beyond the Symposium to build additional support and organization for ongoing action. Obviously, sustaining, expanding and strengthening the work that was started, is essential if meaningful change is to be made. This is done to some extent through a national Interhelp[1] network for despairwork facilitators. However, there is not yet an organized effort to link facilitators and participants with other major groups into a larger social action mode. The ultimate goal of transforming values and structures can come only from sustained effort from many groups over an extended time.

Some vital questions arise. Was the social action an intrusion and improper for a social work conference with a pre-set agenda? Is social action appropriate for social workers and the profession?

Social workers as activists remains problematic and controversial. Though there is a rich tradition dating from Jane Addams and the Settlement House movement, to convert "private troubles into public issues" (Haynes & Mickelson, 1986, p. 6), this has not yet been systematically incorporated into social work methodology. As Grosser points out, "Despite their ultimate vindication, the abolitionist, suffragette and labor organizer are still viewed as historical mutants . . ." (1979, p. 350).

Neutrality of social work may have much to recommend it but has been used to the detriment of certain client groups. With the nuclear arms race, the entire society is the client population at risk in an overriding threat of safety and survival. Carniol (1976) asserts: "Moral outrage at societal conditions needs to be re-introduced into the mainstream of social work practice" (p. 54).

To return to our question: was the action at the Symposium intrusive and improper? Not when one considers that social group work is more aware and attuned to societal needs than other professions, that its educational roots lie in Dewey's participatory democracy

---

[1]Interhelf is a national support network that helps people organize and facilitate programs relating to the planetary dangers of nuclear holocaust, environmental degeneration and human oppression.

and philosophical roots in advocacy and social action. This was most likely why the Symposium participants were receptive to the nuclear workshop spilling over into the luncheon and lobby, not an intrusion at all but a welcome involvement. The author's highlighting of the nuclear issue at other social work meetings, groups generally more concerned with issues of personal growth and change, is now being welcomed where several years ago there was adamant refusal. The profession may now be more receptive to dropping neutrality in the nuclear arms issue and perhaps in others as well.

DIRECTIONS FOR THE FUTURE

The possibility of nuclear annihilation is conceptualized by Lifton as a challenge to the human imagination — "If we can imagine . . . the nuclear holocaust . . . *we can imagine alternatives to that act* (emphasis added) (1982, p. 629). He further asserts: "We are at a moral, biological and imaginative crossroads" (1985).

For mental health professionals, the nuclear threat is a particularly compelling challenge. This population is highly sensitive to quality-of-life issues and responsive where life itself is in peril. It is almost exclusively social workers who facilitate "Changing the Silence" workshops. Presentations at social work settings have brought the most response. The group experience at the Symposium demonstrates the potential for involving the profession. Yet there is currently no major activity in social group work addressing the nuclear danger.

Milton Schwebel (1984), one of the first mental health professionals to speak out on the danger, declares that confronting the nuclear abyss is the work of every "intelligent and enlightened counselor" and not confined to the "radical action of an avant-garde group of counselors" (p. 74). He further asserts that this work "reflects the only direction for ethical practice at this time in the 20th century" (p. 74). It becomes clear that just as we are finally recognizing the AIDS calamity — termed "a health disaster of pandemic proportions" by World Health Organization head Dr. Halfdan Mahler (*N. Y. Times*, 1986) — so we must change our way of thinking about the nuclear threat.

Social group work administrators, educators and others in leadership positions need to explore their individual and agency roles in bringing the nuclear issue to the profession. The profession has a coveted tradition of social action, but unfortunately, leaders, just as others, succumb to numbing mechanisms which obscure this tradition. Social group work presents too lofty a tradition, and the nuclear arms race too ominous a threat, to avoid a constructive confrontation any longer.

There is anxiety in despairwork but the profession has the tools with which to cope. It is clearly and richly endowed with organizational, group and human relation skills to seed its own effort for the survival of the human species. In the past, people could be assured that despite their own deaths, life would continue with future generations. That certainty is now lost. Macy (1983) points out: "That loss, unmeasured and immeasurable, is the pivotal psychological reality of our time" (p. 2). This work may appear to be a grim undertaking, but it is nothing less than a "call to life" (Lifton, 1982, p. 629).

CONCLUSION

The nuclear threat is the ultimate mental health problem. Most individuals, including mental health professionals, ignore this issue. They resort to psychic numbing and reduce themselves to helplessness around this danger. The despair/empowerment workshops help participants lift their numbing and open the possibility for constructive action.

In the Symposium workshop, participants experienced an unusual release of creative energies that were channeled into immediate and concrete action. This experience clearly demonstrates the potency of the despair/empowerment concept and the small-group process. It also suggests that the social group work profession is ready to address the nuclear threat. This is particularly appropriate as a profession concerned with the value of human life.

This work presents a challenge to social group work to discover its mission. The profession embraces a long tradition of social action along with organizational ability and skills to bring to bear on this ominous threat. Lifton urges individuals to go beyond their numbing to challenge their imagination as a "call to life."

REFERENCES

Barnet, R. (1982). Fantasy, reality, and the arms race: Dilemmas of national security and human survival. *American Journal of Orthopsychiatry, 52,* 582-589.

Carniol, B. (1976). The social action process. *The Social Worker, 44*(2-3), 48-54.

Formica, R. (1986). *Leader's guide for love and empowerment in the nuclear age: A workshop approach.* Unpublished manuscript.

Garvin, C. (1984). The changing contexts of social group work practice: Challenge and opportunity. *Social Work with Groups, 7*(1), 18.

Glendinning, C. (1984). The awesome task. *Therapy Now, 1*(2), 10-13.

Glendinning, C. (1987). *Waking up in the nuclear age: A vision for survival.* New York: Beech Tree Books/William Morrow & Co. In press.

Goldman & Greenberg, W. (1982). Preparing for nuclear war: The psychological effects. *American Journal of Orthopsychiatry, 52,* 580-581.

Grosser, C. (1979). Community development programs serving the urban poor. In Compton, B. & Galaway, B. (Eds.). *Social Work Processes* (pp. 345-351). Homewood, Ill.: The Dorsey Press.

Haynes, K. & Mickelson, J. (1986). *Affecting change: Social workers in the political arena.* New York: Longman, Inc.

Intersection Associates (Producer) & Gillingham, M. (Director).(1983). *Changing the silence* Videotape. Boston, Mass. STOP Nuclear War, Inc.

Kieffer, C. (1984). Citizen empowerment: A developmental perspective. In Rappaport, J. & Hess, R. (Eds.). *Studies in empowerment: Steps toward understanding and action* (pp. 9-32). New York: The Haworth Press.

Kübler-Ross, E. (1969). *On death and dying.* New York, Macmillan Publishing Co.

Lifton, R. (1982). Beyond psychic numbing: A call to awareness. *American Journal of Orthopsychiatry, 52,* 619-629.

Lifton, R. (1983). *The broken connection: On death and the continuity of life.* New York, Basic Books/Warner Colophon Edition. Trade edition. Originally published 1969, hardcover edition.

Lifton, R. (1985, February). *Nuclear threat and the problem of imagination.* Paper presented at the meeting of the American Group Psychotherapy Association, New York, N. Y.

Macy, J. (1981). Despair work: *Evolutionary Blues, 1*(1), 36-47.

Macy, J. (1983). *Despair and personal power in the nuclear age.* Philadelphia: New Society Publishers.

McVeigh, K. (1984). *Therapy Now, 1*(2), 24-25.

O'Sullivan, M., Waugh, N., & Espeland, W. (1984). The Fort McDowell Yavapai: From pawns to powerbrokers. In Rappaport, J. & Hess, R. (Eds.). *Studies in empowerment: toward understanding and action* (pp. 73-95). New York: The Haworth Press.

Peck, H. (1984). Do you prefer life to death?: From denial to action. *Transactional Analysis Journal, 14*, 225-228.

Rappaport, J. (1981). In praise of paradox: A social policy of empowerment over prevention. *American Journal of Ccmmunity Psychology, 9*, 1-25.

Schwebel, M. (1984). Growing up with the bomb: Professional roles. *Journal of Counseling and Development, 63*, 73-74.

Teaching Group Work Skill Through Reflection-in-Action

George S. Getzel

SUMMARY. This article explores how social workers with groups think about their practice in the field through insights gathered by instructors using a focused recording device called the "Record of Service." Through the use of this device, social workers are helped to reframe problems as they are experienced by group members and to critically analyze their skill over time. The value of a reflection-in-action epistemology over one that emphasizes technical rationality is argued from findings in records of service.

A perennial question that runs through the discussions and private ruminations of social work educators is: What is the proper division of labor between class and field instructors in the teaching of social work skill? A conventional answer to the question is that in the classroom students are taught scientific theories and principles about practice and in the field the arcane art and wisdom of practice is somehow transmitted. This explanation leaves the "integration" of the science and art of practice to the provenance of the student's mind. While the above is a soothing answer to a perplexing question, it is also a myth which evades the complexity of how students became self-directed and effective learners and social work practitioners.

This paper will try to address the question: How group work practitioners think about practice through findings from a focused

George S. Getzel is a Professor at Hunter College School of Social Work, City University of New York.

instrument that students and teachers can use collaboratively to examine their mutual understandings of ongoing practice problems. The instrument, the Record of Service, is a classroom assignment given to second semester graduate students. The record of service was initially devised under the guidance of the late William Schwartz (1972) of Columbia University for use with agency staff as a tool of accountability to determine if skillful group services were being delivered. Over the last fifteen years the "record of service" assignment has been deepened and elaborated by the author. Students have universally attested that the record of service is a difficult demand, yet it has benefited them greatly in understanding how they work with individuals and groups. Although the record of service is used in the classroom, it is frequently shared by students with their field instructors.

This paper will first describe the mechanics of the record of service as it is introduced to students. Examples of records of service will be used to illustrate the ways students *think* about their group work practice. Finally, the record of service will be examined as it demonstrates and legitimates non-traditional and undervalued ways by which practitioners think about the art or skill of their work with people. Special attention will be given to emerging perspectives of how practitioners think about and evaluate their actions which departs significantly from the ideal of hypothetic deductive logic associated with science and technical rationality (Schön, 1983), *The Mechanics of the Record of Service*.

From the beginning it is crucial that the teacher who uses the record of service emphasizes that it is a device that will help the student think in *new* ways about his or her skill and ongoing practice with groups. The sharing of record of services with the teacher and its presentation to fellow students will be sources of additional insight for the student. The protocols or mechanics of the record of service are meant to help the student enlarge and deepen ways of "seeing" and "reflecting" on practice and are not to be viewed as ends in themselves.

Students are told about records of service over the first few weeks of the semester allowing them to test out problems with a minimum of stress. Students are naturally anxious about exposing their practice errors and shortcomings. The teacher makes clear that the first records of service frequently show very uneven or "bad" practice. While this may be upsetting in the short run, the purpose of the record of service is not to reveal flawless or brilliant skill, but to foster ongoing reflection-in-action—the critical capacity to think about practice as a focused reflection of the worker's understanding of the shifting group process and the worker's contributions to the solutions of group-centered problems. After the record of service demand is carefully spelled out, students begin submitting them to the teacher every two or three weeks.

The following are the steps that the student takes in completing a record of service. The student first reads all process recordings on a group chronologically. The record of service requires doing as complete process recording of verbal and non-verbal content as possible by the student.

The student identifies "problems" *experienced* by the group or by an individual in the group. Problems are not to be identified in terms of symptomatic or personality jargon, but should be understood as the group members experience and understand the identified problem. The student is asked, in short, to imagine through empathy and reflection how a problem he or she sees is felt and understood by group members. This is quite a substantial demand, if taken seriously. Problems thus described are based on some less than superficial description of the relationship of individuals and the group to one another at moments in time.

Each record of service is begun with a face sheet that indicates if it is a group problem or individual problem record of service. Implicit in each statement of a problem are tasks for the social worker which he or she seeks to solve or resolve. It is interesting to note the origin of the word solve come from Latin *solutum*, to loosen. We loosen a problem from its heavy anchorages, but do not necessarily eliminate it. The more complex and serious a problem becomes, the more it needs to be "loosen" as a burden on relevant members. A group problem task for a worker with a group is understood and felt by most members although perceptions and evaluations may differ from member to member. For purposes of doing a group record of service, the student is asked to determine if a problem is predominantly one of the following:

TYPES OF RECORDS OF SERVICE

A. Formation task-problem entails group members' efforts to establish group purpose or contract. It also may be a related question of who is included or excluded from the group.

B. Structure task-problem involves a group's continuing efforts to resolve interpersonal conflicts, decision-making difficulties and related group-wide problem-solving efforts. Some examples of the structural task problems include scapegoating, changing explicit rules or group norms, battles for leadership among individuals and/or sub-groups and so forth. Once again, structural problems are interpersonal and here-and-now concerns.

C. Individual Need Satisfaction Task-problems involve a commonality shared among individuals in the group which periodically confronts members as an issue. The individual need satisfaction task problem encompasses both developmental and situational commonalities such as adolescent members struggling with the potential or the limits of intimacy in relationships with one another or recovering alcoholics handling drinking excesses around Christmas time.

D. Environmental task-problem entails the problems that confront the group from "outside" individuals, primary groups or organizational entities which the membership chooses to deal with as a group. A most common source of environmental problems is the sponsoring agency of the group.

Student Involvement

Individual records of services reflect the worker's and group's task of assisting a particular member with a problem he or she has in the group which arises in the here-and-now of the group or in contexts outside of the group. Examples of this kind of problem include helping a group member with feelings of being rejected by others in the group or assisting a member with strategies which avoid marital fights culminating in violence.

Once the student identifies a specific problem to be examined, he or she excerpts chronologically all process that reflects the problem situation, whether the worker knew of the problem then or not. The student then underlines every intervention that he or she made over any number of sessions. The student is now faced with a collection of skillful and not so skillful interventions, a very unsettling experience to say the least. After thinking simultaneously about the interventions made and what members are experiencing as individuals and members of the group, the worker is asked to state in action terms what the worker *should* endeavor to do with the group or an individual in the group as a reflection of how members experience the particular problem-task. The student is asked to make a summated statement that may serve as a guide to him or herself in evaluating the "rightness" of a pattern of past interventions.

Some examples of problem-task statements are: "To help parents of neo-natal babies in the intensive care unit of a hospital begin to identify and to express more directly their utter sense of helplessness and sense of feeling out of control in regards to the hands-on care of their babies" (an individual need satisfaction type); "To assist aged nursing home residents on a floor to express their suspicions of joining a resident council when they believe that much of the staff and administration of the nursing home has little real interest in them as individuals" (a formation type); "To assist Michael (a member) and the group to sort out his continuing fears, frustrations and actual options in obtaining suitable, safe housing after discharge from a half-way house for recently hospitalized mental patients" (individual type).

After the student is able to write down a relatively clear statement of the problem, he or she has a greater capacity to be productively critical of practice. The student is asked to examine past interventions, and if they are supportive of the problem-task. The student must identify the actual skills used and why the skills were used above dated excerpts of process recordings. It is interesting that the record of service encourages students to deepen their observations and their writing of fuller group process, the source for their analyses and growth as practitioners, A skill list derived from the work Lawrence Shulman (1985) and Lawrence Brammer (1985) is given to students before they prepare record of services.

In the beginning of a record of service, the student supplies relevant facts about the group and members which evolve from the stated problem-task. The student also notes when he or she first became aware of the problem in the group process.

The student completes mini-skill analyses above each unit of dated group process. Process may extend through one or a number of group sessions. Then the student is encouraged in a section labeled, "where the problem stands now" to critically evaluate his or her skill in the sequence of process excerpts. The student is asked to note what was wrong with the practice from the point of view of group members and the student must also look at his or her awareness of what was interfering with his or her use of self.

After critically analyzing the group process and the worker's use of self in the process. the student finds alternative approaches which form "specific next steps" for work with the group and its members. Some future steps may come in the form of cautionary statements to the worker to avoid the impulse to act in a particular way or to try to come in contact with certain affects that worker attaches to different kinds of interaction or characteristics of a particular member. Records of services can be very helpful in locating personal issues for the worker in servicing the needs of members and understanding the underlying processes of the group. Careful distinguishing of self and service requirements is the first step in developing ethically sensitive practice. After completing the formal sequence of thinking about practice or reflection-in-action, the student is asked to list whatever formal concepts or images that occurred to him or her in the course of completing the particular record of service. Concepts may come from the social sciences, humanities or social work practice theory.

Logic of the Record of Service

The record of service serves as a formal structure by which a student can see the artfulness or skill of his or her interventions with a problem experienced by the group. The record of service frames or elucidates the reciprocity of an experienced problem for the group and the worker, and simultaneously depicts the workers' actions over time as he or she experiences them with group members.

The record of services depicts three interpenetrated dimensions of practice 1. the group process in the past influencing the present and pointing to a future; 2. the ongoing understandings of the group process by the worker and group members; and 3. the flow of the worker's actions that purposively and otherwise influence the group process and the worker's and group member's understandings of a problem. The problems of groups reflect the complexity of the interpenetration of all three dimensions as they influence the here-and-now presentation of a problem.

The skill or the art of working with a problem involves the simultaneous joining of perceptions and emotions needed for action to take place. The problems of group and personal existence are unique and complex, and are not subject to direct finite answers, but continuing action.

Philosopher Abraham Heschel (1963), has written

> to ask a question is an act of intellect: to face a problem is a situation involving the whole person. A question is the result of thirst for an answer; a problem calls for a solution. No genuine problem comes into being out of sheer inquisitiveness . . . It comes to pass in moments of being in straits, of intellectual embarrassment, in experiencing tension, conflict and contradiction. To understand the meaning of the problem and to appreciate its urgency, we must keep alive in our reflection the situation of stress and strain in which it comes to pass, genesis and birth pangs, motivation, the face of perplexity, the variety of experiences of it, the necessity of confronting and being preoccupied with it. (p. 11)

Problems seriously faced by a group and worker therefore embody the following:

- emotional tension
- urgency of action
- limits of intellectual understanding
- contradictory or conflicting solutions
- reawakening of past problems and failed efforts (Heschel, 1963)

A CASE ILLUSTRATION

An example of arduous defining process of a problem through reflection-in-action can be seen in a student's record of service description of Maria, a profoundly handicapped thirteen-year-old girl who seemed to court scapegoating from other teenage disabled residents in an intermediate care facility:

> In the fourteenth group session the girls, especially Susan expressed a great deal of hostility to Maria. It was a "positive" occurrence in the group as previous situations of this nature did not surface within the group this blatantly.
>
> Maria comes across as a very frail, helpless, weak, naive and self-pitying early adolescent who angers and in some ways encourages her peers to attack her. Among Maria's strengths is the ability to express her feelings very well and she is open to the viewpoints of others. She can also be very generous and caring, almost to an excess if she detects there is a potential for friendship from a peer.
>
> Maria's family life is very troubled. She has lived with her mother and her mother's numerous male lovers. She and her mother have moved from the South and there is no extended family in the North to help out with Maria's periodic health crises. Maria was born premature with cerebral palsy (spastic diplegia) and walks with the aid of braces and crutches. She is very pretty and fairly independent. However, Maria's mother grows very helpless when she has to deal with Maria's physical needs. Maria's mother blames a series of medical institutions for Maria's health problems. Maria is confused by her mother's neediness and mood swings. Maria implicitly experiences her mother's rejection.
>
> Most of the girls in the group are familiar with Maria's history. She seems to reenact a repulsion attraction pattern with her mother in her relationships with peers. Maria is often attacked by peers in the group. Through looking at relevant process excerpts, I was able to discern a pattern of how Maria

helped in her victimization by group members. It is particularly relevant that this problem has surfaced within the group which prior to open scapegoating of Maria has discussed related group themes — of the hurt and the rejection experienced from peers and family for being disabled and/or having various forms of stigmata.

Despite powerful displays of anger at Maria, group members are able to offer Maria support and concern when she shares personal problems in the group. This is very important to Maria who lacks consistent support from her mother.

Thus, I have begun to see the problem task as my assisting the group to help Maria express her needs for acceptance or approval from others which periodically incurs the wrath of other members (who are possibly upset by similar conflicts of being disabled and rejected). Part of the problem is their use of aggression and their ability to control it. Members need ways to express anger toward Maria which do not debilitate her. Some of the contempt girls feel toward Maria is directly related to her self-pitying behavior. Interestingly, despite all her interpersonal difficulties in the group, she still feels part of the group. The bottom line is that the group still wants to maintain their tie to Maria in the face of these conflicts.

The problem emerges from the group process. With each intervention, the student receives enhanced understanding of the problem's dimensions, while efforts are simultaneously made to solve aspects of the problem. The central characteristic of social work practice is that the means — understanding the problem in-depth is truly inseparable from the end of ameliorating the consequences of the problem. The apportioning of the problems and their solutions can only arise in the complex flux of the group process. As students seek enhanced understanding of the problem, they are often forced to face their own limitations. The graduate student working with Maria and the group writes the following critique of herself in her record of service:

As far as my interventions go, I can generally say that it is hard for me not to jump in when group members are hostile toward Maria. As much as she also can get me angry at times, she makes me very sad and sympathetic. This is something I believe has been transmitted to the other girls and is part of why they are expressive to her, but at the same time seem to care about her.

I have tried to keep my interventions as neutral as possible, although I find this difficult. The amount of anger being expressed scares me. I am afraid that Maria is really going to feel persecuted, misunderstood and abandoned, I find it hard to stay on top of the discussion in my mind when I'm afraid . . . I think I can make a better connection with the topics of sleep, pain, night and death which Maria mentions that upsets the other girls. This might help the group members in their impulse to attack and to shut off Maria. I have to show, even when Maria brings up upsetting topics, careful discussion of what's behind it could be of help with the commonalities of their illness and institutionalization . . . I think when no hostility is on the table, I get very anxious and become a preacher! . . . I can't see that I could continue without investigating this as it boils down to an inability to work with aggressive and hostile feelings, which I know is important to work with.

Through the critique of her work the student is able to see and to approach her work differently in helping the group and Maria. At the end of her enumeration of specific cautions and approaches to working with problems, the student lists the following concepts that illuminated her understanding of the group process, members, interventions and her use of self:

- Scape goating
- Symbiosis
- Separation-individuation
- Self-doubt/pity
- Loss-depression
- Poor self-image
- Needs, fear, wishes

— Projection
— Anger, rage
— Displacement
— Identification
— Empathy
— Cohesion
— Aggression-libido

Richness of theoretical and conceptual resources reflect the considerable skill and understanding available to a student as she reflects-in-action on practice needed to enhance her understanding of the problem and her patterns of intervention.

TOWARD A PRACTICE EPISTEMOLOGY

The logic of the record of service appeals to students of social work practice with groups because, I believe, it reflects the actual ways of knowing and of acting that practitioners use that are neither obfuscated or obscured by the formal teaching of practice which unfortunately gives the assurances and the veneer of science to cover up the intrinsic artfulness of practice.

Lydia Rappaport (1979) in a classic article on "Creativity and Social Work," wrote:

> In social work, the high valuation of the scientific is related largely to our urgent sense of commitment to better fulfill our social purpose in the amelioration and prevention of social ills. It is also related to professional strivings for status and recognition within the framework of our society. In contrast, the creative and the artistic domain of life in society, despite recent artificial and sterile attempts at recognition and elevation, remains outside the pale and is regarded at large with some degree of suspicion. (p. 3)

Science endeavors to provide knowledge to answer questions and the arts attempt to communicate meaning by joining perceptions to emotions. Art or skill is a response or communication emanating from contact with a problem of experience which requires otherwise unavailable perspectives and judgments for effective action to occur.

Donald A. Schön (1983) in a remarkable book, *The Reflective Practitioner*, notes that social workers like practitioners in fields as diverse as management, policy analysis, architecture, and city planning have predicated their continued ability to solve problems on technical rationality. The assumption behind technical rationality is that solutions to practice problems are based on scientifically tested knowledge that rationally explains empirical observations. The argument by some critics is that social work unlike *true* professions such as engineering and medicine is not based on systematic, scientific knowledge which is then applied to successfully solve problems. So-called "true professions" cultivate attitudes among professionals that support the advance of knowledge and do not use techniques or applications which go beyond current scientific knowledge. In short, technical rationality calls for a clear relationship and distinction between means and ends — techniques and intended solutions.

Schön (1983) notes that all professions consequently emphasize their scientific knowledge base and defensively downplay their reliance on artistry or skill in the real world of practice. To focus on artistry or the particularistic aspects of skill would reveal that actions are often taken without a sure or certain understanding of ends or possible outcomes. For the practitioner, means and ends are frequently not known in advance or are even separable. Practitioners often succeed not by knowing in advance or by knowing-in-action, but rather they learn by doing or reflecting-in-action. In the record of service, for example, the student learns about his or her practice by doing and reflecting on the particulars of practice on a specific problem. By then reflecting over on his or her actions and *past* reflections of practice, the student can reframe problems; reanalyze skill and reform his or her practice tendencies. This in-depth reconsideration of practice is not an effort to implement some application of scientific knowledge learned outside of the immediate practice context, but rather an acknowledgement of a reflection-in-action epistemology that arises out of the special circumstances of the here-and-now of practice. Some say this approach is non-conceptual or anti-theoretical. I would disagree but argue that instead of using practice in behalf of theory, the practitioner who is charged with the solution of a problem, is using theoretical insights and concepts that fit the special dictates of the practice situation which cannot be known wholly in advance for a variety of reasons. The discovery of these reasons or circumstances are only possible by taking action in the specific problem context.

IMPLICATIONS

As we all discover sooner or later, professional techniques may generate unforeseen problems and insights that generate requirements for new solutions never considered until then. Examples are numerous – the clinical iatrogenic consequences of a life sustaining drug or the distress other family members experience when the family scapegoat is able to forcefully stand up for himself stepping away from the rewards of enmeshment and punishment.

Very often, professionals are called in when the known and the predictable fail and there are exceptions to the rules. It is not through a positivist epistemology and rationality that much of social work with groups is done. The complexity of individuals, their interactions, group-influenced behavior and even our own well-intended actions preclude a deterministic stance. We group workers instantly experience the emergent every time we enter the exhilarating chaos of group life. Any proffered principle of group intervention must be coached in the conditional, in caveats, and in good humored cautions. It is our cumulative experiences in dealing with the emergent and the unexpected that calls forth our action on the problems in the groups and with individuals. In order to solve problems we not only work with theory and concepts, but with the metaphors of our cumulative or summated experiences in groups and with images stored within our brains that elicit the feelings and tone of our present experience. Middleman and Goldberg (1985) and Lewis (1982) emphasize the importance of these different ways we think about social work practice and group work. The record of service format gives recognition and authenticity to the artful aspects of our practice and different ways of describing our own group experiences.

As important as theory-building about groups is to our knowledge building, developing exemplars of problem depiction and re-flection-in-action live practice is to the cultivation of enhanced skills with groups by social workers. The wider use of records of service and even more importantly the understanding of the record of service's underlying reflection-in-action epistemology has far-reaching consequences for how and what we can teach and learn from our students' work in the field.

William Schwartz (1976) captured the issues of reflection-in-action epistemology:

> The problem that faces the social work profession and other helping disciplines as well, is to describe an art whose achievement depend only partly on the skill of the artist. For until more is known about what goes on in the helping process, social workers will be unable to decide what "it" was that worked and did not . . . to ask the right questions, the major device will for a time remain descriptive, exploratory and theory building, and the primary tool will be the group record, the life history, the critical incident and other techniques for codifying the conceptualizing the experience. (p. 197)

The record of service combines these various modes of understanding practice which is consonant with a reflection-in-action epistemology. Increasingly, we should prepare students to deal with their current practice concerns in the classroom.

REFERENCES

Brammer, L. M. (1985). *The Helping Relation: Process and Skill, Third Edition.* Englewood Cliffs: Prentice Hall.

Heschel, A. J. (1965). *Who Is Man?* Stanford, Calif.: University of Stanford Press.

Lewis, H. (1982). *Intellectual Base of Social Work Practice*, New York: The Haworth Press.

Middleman, R. R. & Goldberg, G. (1985). "Maybe It's a Priest or a Lady with a Hat on It, Or Is It a Bumble Bee?! Teaching Group Workers to See," *Social Work with Groups*, 8(1), Spring, pp. 3-15.

Rappoport, L. (1979). *Creativity and Social Work*, New York: Columbia University Press.

Schön, D. A. (1983). *The Reflective Practitioner: How Professionals Think in Action*. New York: Basic Books.

Schwartz, W. & Serapio, Z. (eds.) (1972). *The Practice of Group Work*, New York: Columbia University Press, pp. 242-265.

Schwartz, W. (1976). "Between Client and System: The Mediating Function," in *Theories of Social Work with Groups*. Roberts, R. W. and H. Northen, eds. New York: Columbia University Press.

Task Group Skills:
The Core of Community Practice

Marie Weil

SUMMARY. This paper will focus on the heart of community practice; work with task groups to improve social conditions and service delivery. Community practice may take place with neighborhood organizations or coalitions, with interagency networks or with coalitions, with interagency networks or with coalitions of volunteers and professionals working toward and advocating for the needs of communities, or special populations, or for particular aspects of social justice and reform.

All community practice is grounded in and carried out through task groups.[1] In social work, task groups may be formed in organizations or communities to plan services, improve service delivery, improve social conditions, empower groups and communities and further social justice. All tasks groups involve planning, decision making and carrying forward actions which will impact on an agency, an inter-organizational network, a community or a special population, The effects of task groups then impact, and are intended always to impact, an environment and social relations beyond the life and interaction of members of the group. Community practice may take place with neighborhood organizations, coalitions or functional communities, through inter-agency networks, or with

Marie Weil, Associate Professor, School of Social Work, The University of Southern California.

1. Note: An expanded version of this paper is Chapter 2 in Weil, M. (in press), *Community practice: Methods, roles and skills*. Homewood, Ill: Dorsey Press.

volunteers and professionals working together for the needs of communities or special populations. It may be focused on general needs or on particular aspects of social justice or reform.

The practice approach needed for work with task groups regardless of interprofessional, citizen or mixed composition requires the staff person or leader to apply methods and skills in a task accomplishment process of mutual planning and decision making. The actions of task groups are, on either a large or small scale, of a political and/or policy development nature. Group planning and decision-making skills are enacted in a political/economic environment. The process in task groups is generic or common with other groups as are some skills, but the focus of the leader or staff person must be on task accomplishment and impact on the external target of change as well as on internal process. This triune focus on decision making and task accomplishment, impact an external target, and internal process renders the role of task group leader different from the roles most typically taken by leaders or therapists with clinical or social development groups.

Students and community practitioners are inevitably engaged in facilitative work with task groups, but are often somewhat disadvantaged in their preparation by a schism between the current literatures (and often curricula) of group work and community organization. Because work with groups over the past two decades has concentrated more and more specifically on clinical/therapeutic intervention models — students may emerge to engage in community practice without knowledge of specific task group aspects of intervention. Indeed they often have to "unlearn" some of the methods and roles which would be natural and unquestioned for a therapist whose primary focus is on the development and growth of members of the groups; and they have to learn for themselves the task facilitation skills of engaging groups in political action or policy planning and implementation.

The community organization literature and curricula through which students would be expected to learn task group methods, on the other hand has been in considerable need of updating to accommodate to changing political, economic and social climates and resources. Much of the best of the community organization literature

(Brager & Specht, 1973; Cox et al., 1877; Cox et al., 1974; Ecklein & Lauffer, 1972; Lauffer, 1978; Kramer & Specht, 1975; Rothman, 1974) was clearly grounded in the practice experience and social/economic climate of the 1960s — a period which current students all too often view as history unrelated to their generation. Recent students have been less and less able to relate to '60s based examples, a situation which reveals that the macro-practice literature on the one hand relied too heavily on specific case tactics and on the other hand made too large a leap between specific example and explanatory theory without providing the needed logic and steps to build practice models and guiding principles to connect cases and theory.

During the later 1970s and early '80s, reflecting economic and social change, there has been a burgeoning of administration literature in social work which has almost eclipsed attention to community organization. The macro-practice literature has become more and more administratively focused on leadership and planning within hierarchies. There has been a decline not only in community organizing foci, but also a decline in literature which deals with agency/citizen joint planning and action, and mutual task group planning.

In both macro- and micro-practice literature and curricula shifts, the focus on task groups has suffered. In micro-practice, therapeutic approaches have nearly eclipsed task approaches; and in macro-practice, hierarchical decision-making processes have taken precedence over mutual decision processes and some of the values of earlier community practice and social work have been displaced.

Three issues need to be dealt with: task group methods and skills need to be clarified; essential values need to be clarified and reintegrated into task group and macro-practice; and macro-practice models need to be updated to reinstate needed community and organizing foci. A recent work edited by Taylor and Roberts (1985) has taken on the challenge of reconceptualizing community practice. This paper builds on the updated models by delineating the core task group skills which are needed to enact the models and reaffirm the values which make community practice a part of social work.

CURRENT MODELS OF COMMUNITY PRACTICE

Taylor and Roberts and their associates (1985) perform a major service for macro-practice by redefining community organization as community practice and by presenting five different models for community practice.

Community development as delineated by Lappin (1985) is focused on local geographic organizing and grounded in an enabling approach which services as both a means to a goal and as a goal itself. This model relates to earlier work by Ross (1955) and to Rothman's (1974) locality development approach.

Program development and coordination incorporates mediative and political processes to bring about implementation of social programs and plans, and develop program coordination. In this model, as articulated by Kurzman (1985), practitioners are primarily involved in work with other professionals and service providers on behalf of the potential service consumers.

Social planning as formulated by Rothman and Zald (1985) has the greatest emphasis on technical skills, formal structures, and research. It concentrates on developing plans and/or forecasting conditions and developing plans intended to be logical, rational, and beneficial for a specific population or area.

Community liaison is the most recently defined model of community practice. Taylor (1985) develops this model to represent an holistic approach at the individual agency level to integrate social work roles in both environmental and interpersonal change processes. This model specifies community practice/liaison roles for multiple levels of staff and administrators of direct service agencies which are tied to the purposes and goals of the agency.

Pluralism, participation, and political empowerment. This model as defined and developed by Crosser and Mondros (1985) builds on earlier social action models. It focuses on increasing participation and power of groups who have been excluded from decision processes in order to achieve their self-defined, desired goals. It is grounded in the realities of struggle and the existence of conflicting interests in any community.

These five models greatly enrich macro-practice and define the field of community practice in a much more discrete and comprehensive manner. In order to effectively incorporate these models into curricula and practice it is important to clarify essential issues in value orientation and to specify the generic task group facilitation skills which are necessary to enact and give life to the models.

VALUES FOR COMMUNITY PRACTICE

As recent history in the political and legal fields gives abundant testimony, professional values are as much needed in macro-practice arenas as they are in therapeutic treatment. Values not only inform the choices of practice interventions and strategies but are the element of community practice which maintains its connection with the field of social work. Organizing and planning are processes which can as easily, or more easily, be used for oppression and destruction as for empowerment. It is critical to define the central values of community practice which determine the nature of the relationship between the professional and group and which shape chosen goals and strategies.

Clarification of values can indeed be one means to reclaim and revitalize social work's involvements with and commitment to community practice. Direct community organization and voluntary social action as basic methods of social work practice have been muted by declining funding, diminished resources and changing modes of practice. Much of the early community social work literature (for example Ross, 1955) focused strongly on values and highlighted the importance of process, group facilitation and democratic participation. The trends in micro- and macro-practice noted earlier, particularly the increasing technocratic focus on many administrative models and the subsuming of much group and community practice into generic orientations have for different reasons deemphasized the values critical for community practice. As values material was written for generic curricula, the phrasing and examples most often related to micro-practice of clinical concerns. The administrative literature when it treated values related more to hierarchical connections to employees and to ministerial relations to clients. Much of the later community organization literature moved toward increased specialization. It highlighted theoretical and ideological differences in approaches and emphasized specialized analytic models and strategies without concomitant emphasis on values, processes and skills common to all community practice.

The common grounding of values, process and skills for community practice needs to be clarified and stressed in the education of students and the training of practitioners. With all social workers, community practitioners should subscribe to the established professional values based on individual dignity and social interdependence (Dromi & Weil, 1984).

In addition to those basic values, all social workers: clinicians, administrators, and planners as well as community organizers should be grounded in central community practice values of participation, social justice, and social responsibility. These values shape ethical practice and guide development of practice principles and intervention strategies.

Participation as a value and principle for community practice implies citizen and worker involvement in community and organizational decision-making. Participation emphasizes democratic structuring. It implies inclusiveness, attention to divergences and efforts toward consensus building. Brager and Specht (1973) delineated the tensions inherent in values of participation, expertise and leadership. However leadership can be construed collectively and as shared, and expertise can be taught. In community practice, expertise and leadership should be engaged to increase and enable democratic participation. Freire (1981) offers models through which even illiterate and oppressed groups can be engaged in analysis and action to increase participation. Burghardt (1983) offers means of working with union members and other groups toward participatory empowerment. Weil (1985) discusses principles of democratic structuring and empowerment as part of a feminist reconceptualization of community practice.

Social Justice. As a value and a principle, social justice implies analysis and action toward eliminating racism, sexism, discrimination, oppression and exclusion of disadvantaged groups and vulnerable populations from social and political involvements. It speaks to the social work responsibility to actively engage against oppressive structures and to work with vulnerable groups, with those in power, and with service systems to achieve a more equitable, humane and just society. Commitment towards social justice involves a commitment to developing social institutions which respect individual, group, and inter-group civil rights and social and economic opportunities. For social work clinicians as well as community workers, the professional value for promoting social justice involves commitment to case and class advocacy. As Rothman (1971) notes, holding the value of social justice mandates a commitment to disadvantaged racial and ethnic groups to assure services and to develop appropriate service and community support models (Weil, 1981). The political empowerment model (Grosser & Mondros, 1985) is grounded in support for social justice, and the community development model (Lappin, 1985) moves toward social justice and increased participation for the disadvantaged. Grosser and Mondros (1985) note that in order to achieve goals of empowerment, previously excluded or disadvantaged groups may establish their own community based services.

Social responsibility as a value for community practice articulates the social interdependence of all people and highlights the professional responsibility to act in ways to define and clarify that interdependence for groups, communities, programs, social institutions, and societies. The profession of social work is about social responsibility. Community practice is the most direct means of acting on that social responsibility to humanize social institutions, to open up the political process, and to insure social action aimed at human survival. This value embodies the ethical responsibility to act to protect the vulnerable, to act in ways that express mutual interdependence and to value and support the needs of the disadvantaged. Enacting the value of social responsibility ranges from seeing that a client receives a needed service, to conducting research to document changing patterns of vulnerability, developing and implementing policy to combat racism and sexism, to social action in support of oppressed groups, to action to assure a nuclear free future and the future of humanity.

Translation of these values into principles shapes practice. Action on value based principles requires practice skills in task group facilitation. Professional commitment to social justice and advocacy can be carried forward through the work of task groups engaged in dealing with the problems of communities, oppressed groups and vulnerable populations. Regardless of the scale of a community practice project, whether it is a small inter-agency team, a large citizen organization, or a citizen/agency coalition — its working units are invariably small groups or subgroups such as committees or task forces involved in the definition, strategic planning, decision-making and accomplishment of particular tasks. Large organizations like large social movements rely on sub-groups to handle specified responsibilities and actions. Task groups then are the heart of community practice and the means through which the goals of community interventions are accomplished. The targets of task group change may be a community, an organization or service system, or a society. In order to impact these targets the members of task groups must be able to engage in concerted collaborative processes. Practitioners require specific skills to enable collaboration processes. Practitioners require specific skills to enable collaboration and decision-making.

TASK GROUP SKILLS FOR COMMUNITY PRACTICE

Work with inter-and intra-professional teams, service planning groups, interagency task forces, research groups, community groups, citizens organizations and social action movements all require task group practice skills. Regardless of the type of task group or the organizational level of the professional, a generic set of tasks group practice skills are essential: 1. task group development and facilitation, 2. direct leadership and leadership development, 3. organizing, 4. planning, 5. provision of information and expertise, and 6. empowerment.

TASK GROUP DEVELOPMENT AND FACILITATION

The work of developing a task group for community practice may range from knocking on doors in a neighborhood to ascertain if people are interested in street lights, traffic signs or local education issues or selecting and engaging people to plan and organize a political action campaign, to convening a case management contract meeting among service providers for developmentally disabled clients, to convening agency directors to develop a pro-active stance with regard to policy proposals or collaborative service agreements.

To develop a group, the worker must know what the issue is (or be willing to accept issues identified by citizens) and must decide who to contact about involvement and how to contact them. Skill in group development relates to strong understanding of group dynamics and factors in group composition such as homogeneity, diversity, relative power, ability to collaborate, and willingness to commit to specified tasks. Creating a group or deciding who to invite may well be a very difficult part of a community practice process.

Facilitating the participation and decision-making of group members requires high levels of skill regardless of the sophistication of the members. Initially the facilitator as formal or informal leader must establish a climate for meetings which fosters trust, encourage people to share their concerns, and enable the group to develop a common ground for action, Developing that ability to share may require individual meetings or phone conversations with prospective members. Early efforts to draw out members' interests and commonalities and indicate where concerns are shared can build positive expectations of participating in a task group process. Skills in facilitating process and task accomplishments undergird all other group skills.

Basic skills in facilitation include the following:

1. *Establishing Clarity of Purpose.* The facilitator must be able to help the group come to a consensus regarding its purpose and tasks. The more specific the goals and steps to achieve them can be delineated, the clearer the groups' activities will become (Ross, 1955).
2. *Developing a Climate of Attention and Considerations.* The facilitator must be able to listen to group members and draw out their ideas (Toseland & Rivas, 1984). Basic skills in instrumental leadership are the issue. The facilitator may need to ask quieter members about their ideas or modify the flow of discussion so that all with an opinion have a chance to express it.
3. *Reframing and Integrating Ideas.* Facilitation skills are often required in restating or reframing comments or ideas. The facilitator may need to defuse language and interpret ideas from

one member to another. She or he may need to show how the ideas of group members complement or diverge from each other, and frequently may need to restate ideas to clarify them and be sure of the intended meaning.

4. *Assess the Consensus Building and Decision Making Process.* Facilitators need to ascertain in formal or informal ways whether the group members are in agreement about an idea or a proposed action (Toseland & Rivas, 1984). This may range from looking at the members, scanning for reactions (Middleman, 1978), to asking if anyone dissents, to asking for a vote. Where there is disagreement, the skilled facilitator will try to at least clarify and specify the areas of disagreement and ascertain what the disagreement means for the work of the group. The facilitator may need to work with the group to develop alternative strategies or even to change the focus or purpose of the task group.

5. *Develop Inclusiveness.* Facilitators often have to assure that ideas of lower status, token, or newer members of a group are noticed. Building a climate which supports participation and democratic structuring may become a central task (Weil, 1985). The facilitator often leads in developing patterns of responding to the ideas and proposals of members. Assisting members in developing, "owning," and evaluating ideas is a central facilitation function.

6. *Enact Democratic Leadership.* Depending on whether the facilitators are formal leaders, i.e., chairperson of a group or staff to the group, they will need to take on role appropriate behavior in expressing their own ideas. The autocratic chairperson or staff is frequently the death of a group or at least of commitment to the group's purpose. Yet a non-committal leader can also be damaging to group moral and decision making.

7. *Model Positive Communication and Supportive Feedback.* Facilitators need to model and nurture positive communication patterns among group members, Clarifying statements, reframing or interpreting ideas, and acknowledging contributions as well as providing supportive comments and maintaining task focus contribute to a positive communication climate.

8. *Guide Interaction.* Directly or indirectly facilitators frequently need to guide group discussion and patterns of interaction. The metaphor often used for this process is orchestrating a meeting. Within task groups, it is important to have a facilitator who can keep people on track, keep focused on needed decisions, and balance that orientation to attend to process issues and problems. Hurrying a decision may well result in lack of commitment; prolonging decision making and action may result in loss of the more committed members.

9. *Balance Process and Tasks.* Facilitators must assist a group in balancing its process and task orientations, assure that both are attended to and make certain that process issues are integrated into task accomplishment.

Task Group Leadership and Leadership Development

In work with neighborhood groups, functional community groups or interagency task forces, it is important to clarify whether the professional serves as staff, as a formal leader or as a developer of leadership. In the types of community groups discussed by Twelvetrees (1976) and the community development model described by Lappin (1985), leadership development is the worker's central task. Often one of the initial problems is clarifying with formal leaders the distinctions between formal leadership responsibilities and staff responsibilities (Weil, 1967). For most task groups associated with social work programs, autocratic or authoritarian models of leadership are not desirable. If goals in work with citizens and/or staff are to develop leadership, then acceptance of responsibility and decision-making abilities must be nurtured. For many groups whether they are citizens in a block club, representatives in a federation of neighborhood groups, or staff members, a model of democratic, functionally shared leadership is preferable to reliance on position power (Weil, 1967). Viewing leadership as the ability to mobilize people and resources, to get things done, to provide expertise, and to influence the attitudes and behaviors of others can be handled so that the function of leadership is shared or rotated depending on the expertise required for a particular issue, Matrix management models acknowledge this possibility. Groups which have sound respect for members' abilities can often foster patterns of shared leadership which are functional in achieving goals, and positive forces for growth and adult development in the lives of group members.

As a leader, the worker models leadership functions in facilitating, planning and decision making. When involved in leadership development, the worker will need to assist group members in managing meetings, preparing agendas, planning ways to facilitate communication, examining ways to move toward decision making, balancing task and process concerns, analyzing influence and opportunities, and evaluating the progress of the group and skill development of the leaders. Newer group members will need to be trained for leadership and participation and may need to take on leadership functions incrementally.

Typically in community practice, the worker will fulfill leadership roles as an enabler—that is "helping the group to acquire needed information or resources, to determine its priorities and procedures, and to plan a strategy for action" (Toseland & Rivas, 1984). As Grosser and Mondros (1985) point out, the worker may provide direct leadership functions in such tasks as lobbying or needs assessment research.

Directive roles are risky in that group members may become dependent on staff to handle public relations or advocacy. Leadership development is extremely important in this area and the worker can train and enable group members in advocacy, public relations and media contact skills so that the group can learn to act autonomously in its external relations as its internal operations (Abels, 1980). Assisting members in asking questions and testing the consequences of decisions can help build autonomy within the group.

Basic skills for leadership development include:

1. Assisting group members in identifying their own abilities.
2. Modeling leadership tasks such as balancing task and process in group meetings and decision making.
3. Helping group members learn to locate and use information and resources.

4. Assisting group members in conducting needed research and teaching them research utilization skills.
5. Enabling and training members to develop skills in public relations and media encounters.
6. Assisting members in evaluating their own process, their progress toward goal accomplishment and constraints.
7. Coaching group members in consensus building, decision making, and advocacy skills.
8. Coaching members in strategies for dealing with internal and external conflict and assisting them in analyzing, selecting, and implementing educational, collaborative, contest, and adversarial strategies (Brager & Specht, 1973).
9. Helping members question strategies and design fall-back positions or secondary strategies.
10. Clarifying roles, supporting members in making their own decisions, without concealing own views.

ORGANIZING

Organizing is both an interactional and a technical process. It involves identification, selection, and mobilization of resources and selection and mobilization of people for involvement in strategies for change. A major area of staff facilitation in organizing is in clarifying roles which group members will play in a particular project or change process as well as assisting group members in identifying and sequencing tasks, and assigning responsibility for task and goal accomplishment.

Organizing relates to setting goals and developing an action plan with carefully orchestrated steps, It requires carrying plans forward and evaluating outcomes.

The worker may well be closely involved in action plans but needs to treat the process as an educational, training and empowerment process for group members. Helping members "rehearse" their roles in a change or social action strategy is one particularly useful means of skill development and consolidation.

Basic skills in organizing include:

1. Assisting the group in analyzing a problematic situation and determining an action approach.
2. Assisting the group in mapping out an action strategy.
3. Determining needed resources, roles, and tasks to effect change.
4. Scheduling and organizing people and resources to carry out change strategies and social action.
5. Assisting the group in orchestrating the change process.
6. Working with the group to evaluate the change process and define next steps.

Planning

Planning is the process of analyzing problems, determining possible alternatives, forecasting consequences and choosing preferred actions and outcomes. Planning processes frequently involve using technical research skills, and teaching others to use them. In working with community groups, the worker may function as an advocate planner, or enabler and trainer for the group.

Basic planning skills include:

1. Conducting research and needs assessments and teaching group members these methods.
2. Assisting groups in learning community research procedures, and skills in utilizing research results.
3. Assessing the group and its environment.
4. Delineating possible outcomes and anticipating "unanticipated consequences."
5. Recommending most feasible courses of action to deal with a particular issue.
6. Documenting and evaluating plan implementation and results.

PROVISION OF INFORMATION AND EXPERTISE

In the course of planning and organizing, the worker frequently must provide a group with information, help them to determine what information they need and educate or train them to carry out this function themselves (Grosser & Mondros, 1985: Weil, 1985).

In lending expertise, the worker should also take on a training role to assist the group members in gaining expertise needed to carry out their goals. Expertise may be technological and/or interactional. Critically, however, in order to impart expertise, one must have it.

Basic skills in developing expertise in a group include:

1. Sharing information.
2. Assisting the group in analyzing the skills they need to develop.
3. Offering assistance in skill development in a manner that builds confidence and empowers members of the group.
4. Assisting group members in identifying resources for further learning and knowledge and skill development.

Empowerment

Empowerment is an educational, consciousness raising process which enables people to deal with obstacles and problems, to exert leadership and to increase decision-making power in their lives and communities (Solomon, 1985, 1976). Where community practice is not focused on empowerment, it betrays its central purpose to help people help themselves. Empowerment models place the professional in the service of the self-defined needs of oppressed troubled communities and groups (Grosser & Mondros, 1985). Empowerment approaches prepare the oppressed or disadvantaged to analyze and understand community problems, plan remedies and work toward solutions. Such approaches emphasize demystifying power and expertise and develop means for sharing both (Weil, 1985). Empowerment models envision shared leadership and expertise and are grounded in the value of participation.

Integrating Skills and Values

Skills in these six areas serve as the foundation for practice in any community intervention approach. They are pivotal in helping a group to define priorities, develop action plans, develop consensus building and problem solving strategies and carry action forward. These skills enable the community practitioner to focus on both task and process components of task group facilitation. They assist in reclaiming the historical focus on democratic participation in community practice, and reintegrate central values of commitment to social justice and social responsibility into community practice. Because these skill areas can effectively unite professional values and sound principles of practice, they should be incorporated in all community practice and teaching models.

Recent concentration on technological skills in community practice has displaced the centrality of these basic task group practice skills. They need to be restored to their pivotal place in the education and training of community practitioners at direct service, planning, community organization and administrative levels. These skills are generic across community practice models and constitute the basic practice armamentarium required for effective work within task groups. With these basic skills in place, workers can mere easily master model-specific and macro-focused skill areas. They will also be better able to utilize their technical skills in group processes. While the models of community practice (Taylor & Roberts, 1985) frequently require special expertise and the use of contest and adversarial strategies in their work to affect external targets of change, the collaborative, group development approach which is an outgrowth of application of the six core skills described here is essential to enable task groups to develop the cohesion, clarity and commitment to affect social, community and organizational change. Without careful development of the task group itself through supportive and empowering strategies, the group will not be effective in action. Unless practitioners have competence in these central task group process skills, much of community practice will fall short of its goal to involve professionals and citizens in work and advocacy for community development, political action, organizing, planning and empowerment.

REFERENCES

Abels, P. (1980). Instructed advocacy and community group work. In A. Alissi (Ed.). *Prospectives on social group work practice*. New York: The Free Press, 326-331.

Brager, G.A. & H. Specht (1973). *Community organizing*. New York: Columbia University Press.

Burghardt, S. (1982). *The other side of organizing*. Cambridge, Mass.: Schenkman.

Cox, F.M., J.L. Erlich, J. Rothman, & J.E. Tropman (Eds.) (1974). *Strategies of community organization*. Itasca, Ill.: F.E. Peacock.

Cox, F.M., J.L. Erlich, J.Rothman, & J.E. Tropman (Eds.) (1977). *Tactics and techniques of community organization*. Itasca, Ill: F.E. Peacock.

Dromi, P. & M. Weil (November, 1984). Social group work values: Their role in a technological age. Paper presented at the Sixth Annual Symposium for the Advancement of Social Work with Groups. Chicago.

Ecklein, J.L. & A.A. Lauffer (1972). *Community Organizers and Social Planners*. New York: John Wiley and Sons.

Freire, P. (1981). *Pedagogy of the Oppressed*. New York: Continuum.

Grosser, C.F. & J. Mondros (1985). Pluralism and participation: The political action approach. In S.H. Taylor and R.W. Roberts (Eds.). *Theory and Practice of Community Social Work*. New York: Columbia University Press, 154-178.

Kramer, R.M. & H. Specht (Eds.) (1975). Readings in community organization practice: Second Edition. Englewood Cliffs, N.J.: Prentice-Hall.

Kurzman, P.A. (1985). Program development and service coordination as components of community practice. In S.H. Taylor and R.W. Roberts (Eds.). *Theory and practice of community social work*. New York: Columbia University Press, 95-124.

Lappin, B. (1985). Community development: Beginnings in social work enabling. In S.H. Taylor and R.W. Roberts (Eds.). *Theory and practice of community social work*. New York: Columbia University Press, 59-94.

Lauffer, A. (1978). *Social planning at the community level*. Englewood Cliffs: N.J.: Prentice-Hall.

Middleman, R. (1978). Returning group process to group work. *Social Work with Groups*, Vol. 1(10), 15-26.

Ross, M.G. (1955). *Community organization: Theory and principles*. New York: Harpers.

Rothman, J. (1974). *Planning and organizing for social change*. New York: Columbia University Press.

Rothman, J. (Ed.) (1971). *Promoting social justice in the multigroup society*. New York: Association Press.

Rothman, J. & M.N. Zald (1985). Planning theory in social work community practice. In S.H. Taylor and R.W. Roberts (Eds.). *Theory and practice of community social work*. New York: Columbia University Press, 125-153.

Solomon, B.B. (1976). *Black empowerment: Social work in oppressed communities*. New York: Columbia University Press.

Solomon, B.B. (1985). Community social work practice in oppressed minority communities. In S.H. Taylor and R.W. Roberts (Eds.). *Theory and practice of community social work*. New York: Columbia University Press, 217-257.

Taylor, S.H. (1985). Community work and social work: The community liaison approach. In S.H. Taylor and R.W. Roberts (Eds.). *Theory and practice of community social work*. New York: Columbia University Press, 179-214.

Taylor, S.H. & R.W. Roberts (Eds.) (1985). *Theory and practice of community social work*. New York: Columbia University Press.

Toseland, R.W. & R.F. Rivas (1984). *An introduction to group work practice*. New York: MacMillan.

Twelvetrees, A.C. (1976). *Community associations and centres: A comparative study*. Oxford: Pergamon.

Weil, M. (1967). Leadership building as a community development process. Master Thesis, University of Pennsylvania, School of Social Work.

Weil, M. (1981). Southeast Asians and Service Delivery, in *Bridging cultures*. Los Angeles: Asian American Community Mental Health Training Center.

Weil, M. (1985). Women, community and organizing. In N.Van Den Bergh and L.B. Cooper (Eds.). *Feminist visions for social work*. Silver Spring Md.: National Association of Social Workers.

Staff Groups: Creative Problem-Solving in the Workplace

Leonard N. Brown

Faced with increasing labor and health costs in this country and sharper competition from abroad, American management is overhauling the corporate structure. The basis for much of their redesign is the use of the worker to solve workplace problems (Naisbitt, 1984; Serrin, 1984). Part of the revolution in business practices is quality circles, an import from Japan, in which small groups of employees meet to suggest improvements in their work processes and products. It is estimated that over 90% of the Fortune "500" companies now use quality circles (Lawler & Mohrman, 1985). Businesses and industries are discovering that their most important resource is the employee, a largely untapped source of strength for improving the quality of work life. The "bottom line" for justifying the expense of removing employees from their work stations to participate in problem-solving activities is that it has reduced company costs. Some of the savings comes from a reduction in burnout and less stress from the fallout of a depersonalized work situation (Jackson & Schuler, 1983).

Together with this trend has been the movement toward "wellness programs" in the corporate sector. Management has recognized that workers who are healthier will be an asset to their performance and their place of work. Ironically, human service organizations, which might be expected to be the first to recognize the worth of the individual and value of the small group, have been slow to initiate the

Leonard N. Brown, Professor, School of Social Work, Rutgers University, 536 George Street, New Brunswick, New Jersey 08903.

wellness concept. Stress and associated burnout are rampant in social agencies (Brown, 1984; Cherniss, 1980). The focus of this paper is to discuss the use and value of staff support and problem-solving groups in human service organizations. This paper assumes that this approach will accomplish the dual goals of personal fulfillment and improved work productivity.

THE INDIVIDUAL, GROUP AND ORGANIZATION

The literature from small group theory suggests that groups engaged in cooperative activities are generally more successful than are competitive groups. This has been demonstrated in terms of closer work relationships, higher morale, and the ability to complete complex tasks and increase productivity. Cooperative groups have the potential of meeting the needs of both individuals and the organization (Tjosvold, 1984). Systems theory, which discusses how parts of a system that are strengthened contribute to the growth of the larger system, may also be used as a conceptual rationale for the use of small cooperative groups within organizations. The concept of systemic linkage, more specifically, is that two parts of a system create a more powerful union than when each part acts separately.

Another theoretical link to support employee involvement is the notion of expressivism as a dimension of Maslow's hierarchy of needs. The levels that Maslow describes include the satisfaction of physiological needs, safety needs, belongingness and social needs, egoistic needs and self-actualization needs. Expressivism is mostly related to the fulfillment of these higher order needs, such as fulfilling egoistic needs and reaching self-actualization (Yankelovich, 1983). McGregor's "Theory Y" is a further justification for elevating the worth and dignity of the employee so that the work environment becomes more conducive for growth of the individual and organization. Theory Y assumes that workers want to exercise responsibility, become more creative and actually use their intellect more fully. Ineffective work performance is only partially related to the functioning of the employee. In this model the organization becomes deficient if it is not able to design a way of using individual and group capacities for growth and change (Barra, 1983).

ORGANIZING STAFF GROUPS

A hospital* was the host setting for a training and research project to establish problem-solving staff groups. These groups, meeting voluntarily on work time, were designed to accomplish the following:

1. Act as a support and resource group for each of the members.
2. Provide an opportunity to explore alternative responses and attitudes about themselves, job stress and their co-workers.
3. Enable group members to learn appropriate knowledge and skills of problem-solving.
4. Recommend action plans to implement their suggestions within the organization.

Groups from high stress work areas, such as nurses and social workers from oncology and interdisciplinary staff from a brain trauma unit, were initially recruited for the groups. Other nurses from middle and upper level management also agreed to participate in the group program. Each of the four groups started with about ten members.

One of the unique features of these groups is that the leaders were chosen by the group from within their ranks. It is expected that in this situation all participants would be more willing to risk the sharing of personal experiences. The peer leader can offer a less threatening form of leadership than can a supervisor. Hopefully, this type of person will be more empathetic than a supervisor since he or she is experiencing a similar situation. We recognize that there is an informal social system in any organization with a ranking of persons who exercise different types of leadership. The peer system can be a powerful influence in shaping values and behavior. In this case we are "tapping into" this informal system and formalizing the indigenous leadership. In this way these groups resemble self-help groups with more of a task-oriented emphasis. The leaders participate in a series of initial training workshops on group dynamics and skills. These sessions are followed by ongoing training to discuss progress and problems in the groups. In this way the

---

*John F. Kennedy Medical Center, Edison, New Jersey.

leaders receive continued support and skill development in their role as facilitators.

A FRAMEWORK FOR GROWTH AND CHANGE

The training of the leaders emphasizes a framework for growth and change as a foundation for a problem-solving approach with the groups. It is assumed that if the leaders could understand the multiple facets of a change process, they would make better use of helping skills.

To illustrate the meaning of these concepts more fully, excerpts from one session of the oncology group will be given for each part of the framework. This group is composed of nurses and social workers. Two nurses were chosen by the group to be facilitators. The group had been meeting for a month at the time of this particular session.

1. Identification and Clarity of the Problem of Need

Reaching consensus about a problem or need affecting group participants is the first step toward resolution. The interaction of group members to achieve clarity about their reasons for meeting is the beginning of a bond of closeness. It is really the first task of the group. Being able to separate the problem into manageable parts makes the eventual problem-solving more attainable. The group sets priorities for action by considering which parts are most accessible to change.

In the group a nurse discusses the problem of insufficient staffing of nurses on the oncology floor.

> We have to start recognizing the problems that we face. That's reality. A lot of people say we don't have short staff. Being short staffed on the floor where the patients can walk and eat and talk and take showers for themselves is a lot different than being in a facility where these patients can't do much for themselves. We're responsible. The blame always comes to us if the patient hasn't eaten, hasn't been washed, bed changed, medication isn't on time. What about giving us a little break and saying we understand and try to get something accom-

plished from this. Let's get the staffing in there that will give the patients better care.

In this case the group recognizes a rather global problem. The group members perceive the problem as existing outside of the group and in the hands of the administration for resolution. It is very natural for people to conceptualize a problem as having its source somewhere else. Where this happens the possibilities for solution become more nebulous and distant as the problem is further removed from those persons who have identified it in the first place.

2. Favorable Conditions and Environment

Too often the conditions for learning or change are overlooked. It may be assumed that if participants are having problems, it is all internal—within the person. We now recognize that the environment can enhance or impede growth. Within any organization there may be insufficient resources for staff to function successfully in their jobs. Communication may be inadequate or there may be mixed messages, a source of confusion in any interaction. Role expectations may be unclear or unreasonable. Supervisory help may be unavailable or inadequate for the particular needs of the staff person. When these kinds of problems exist the staff group will need to use its internal strength as a constructive environment to identify organizational issues for resolution. Together the group should be able to engage appropriate persons in the workplace who are in a position to make the necessary changes toward a more favorable climate of work.

In this case the group itself becomes the constructive environment for change:

> I didn't realize I was under so much stress until the last month or so, until we actually started having these meetings. A lot of things are coming out now that I didn't realize about myself and right now I'm dealing with it better by coming to these meetings every Thursday and it seems to be helping more. Just by being able to talk and let other people listen to what I am feeling and know that they care about what I am saying.

3. Necessary Knowledge and Skills

The giving and receiving of information that is related to a topic under discussion is a necessary part of planning further steps. Group members may be able to offer appropriate help, or it may be necessary to seek additional resources from persons outside the group, such as supervisors or staff with responsibilities for an area of the hospital. This is also true of skill development, for which the Department of Training and Education could be available. This part of the framework emphasizes that staff take more control and responsibility for their own learning. They become proactive in defining their needs and in seeking the resources for accomplishing their goals. The use of the group is particularly helpful in making it possible for them to succeed. The fact is that a group of people, working together and seriously deliberating about an issue, lends power and credibility to their request. The involvement of supervisory staff is essential so that the administrative structure is operational.

The nurses and hospice counseling staff (Haven) work on the same floor with the patients and their families. Prior to the group meetings, their relationship was strained. One of the nurses discusses how knowledge about the hospice program has helped them all in working more closely together.

> I think it has opened a great deal of communication between all of us because we were not aware of what Haven was doing. I wasn't aware of problems that you had and I'm sure that you weren't totally aware of the problems we had.

4. Recognition of Attitudes and Feelings

Staff often want to share their attitudes and feelings with colleagues who are willing to listen and understand. Being able to engage in dialogue can provide employees with the necessary support and recognition to manage job stress and work toward feasible solutions. It is not enough for the staff groups to be task-centered or goal-directed. Developing positive attitudes and feelings can change perceptions in a more hopeful direction. The staff's self-perceptions and feelings can affect their relationships with patients and how they administer care.

Before I used to go home and say, well I put in my 8 hours and this is just a job and that's how I treated it. But I didn't realize how much stress I was having until you started to talk in here and you know it just kind of opened itself up and a lot of things were being released now that I didn't think I had inside. I thought I was this real tough person that came in here every day to put in 8 hours and that was it.

Some of the denial experienced by this nurse may have been necessary for her in warding off overwhelming feelings of anxiety. She needed to be able to function in her job. However, stress can often produce symptoms of physical and emotional disturbance. It is likely that the nurse was able to give up this defense mechanism of denial as she was able to receive the support from others in the group. Recognition of the feelings associated with the stress makes it more possible to deal with the strain constructively. The nurse is able to realize that others are facing a similar situation and can lend their resources to the solution of the problem. In their collective wisdom the group members are able to identify varied sources of the stress, hopefully partializing aspects of the problem so that some areas become more manageable for solutions. Some of the change may take place in how the nurse perceives the problem. In the ensuing discussion she is able to gain new insights into the meaning of work stress for her and to develop an approach to deal with it that becomes less self-abusive.

5. Initiative Toward Action

In the initial training of group leaders and subsequent ongoing consultation, a strong value was placed on developing action plans. Too often group members meet for the purpose of raising issues or expressing feelings without doing anything toward resolution. Taking action involves a risk. The plan may be rejected or it may not succeed if adopted. If the prior steps have been followed so that the group has access to relevant data and can express feelings in a comfortable and constructive manner, it is likely that action will follow as a natural step toward problem-solving. When the group is planning action, it should consider the feasibility of recommendations, setting priorities and the possibilities of joining with others who share common goals. Part of what staff groups need to focus upon are areas that are within their control. The attempts to make sweeping changes within the hospital may be a way of resisting the more obvious problems within their own group environment, such as relationships among the group members, changes in procedures within their work areas or sharing of pertinent information about patients to improve care.

In attempting to resolve the problem of insufficient staff during a crisis on the floor, the group members discuss a possible solution:

Social Worker: But what kind of help could you get on such sudden notice? It wouldn't be someone trained for this unit.

Nurse: We have floats all the time that come to our floor and make us still short but at least we are going to get out at a reasonable hour. The patients are going to get a decent amount of care. There's no reason why if another floor is less critical, it's really not that important to have that 5th or 6th nurse there. It is really that important to us — what we're doing is usually with more critical patients, not always the only critical ones but on an average our patients are more critical. Realize that it is very bad. Realize that that patient may need one-on-one care for the entire shift.

Social Worker: So if the supervisor could make that judgment it would be up . . .

Nurse: It would be up to the supervisor to send someone.

Social Worker: Then the administration should trust that supervisor's judgment. If she says it has to be that way, it does.

All aspects of the framework are essential to create a state of wellness. Depending upon the group, its composition, purpose and stage of development, some areas will be emphasized more than others. The model also has assessment value in detecting strengths and deficiencies in how groups are attempting to solve problems.

LEVELS OF PROBLEM-SOLVING WITHIN THE HOSPITAL

There are three levels of problem-solving that can take place in the workplace. The staff group is the basic unit to enhance growth and productive change. The group members are able to experience additional control and responsibility for their lives. They are able to recognize and use personal strengths as well as the many varied resources within the group. The interaction within the group can have an energizing effect on the participants, as they are able to receive recognition and acceptance for their ideas. The group can also be helpful in testing the reality and feasibility of ideas. If some proposals for change are "too far out," the wisdom of collective thinking will often produce a more practical avenue to success. People become more aware of the power of positive thinking and use of constructive attitudes in dealing with what may seem like insurmountable obstacles. Having the tools of problem-solving available is another way that group members can systematically work on finding alternatives to deal with difficult situations. Finally, the group can produce the energy, creativity and momentum to move ideas to a level of constructive action. It is expected that action will take place in relation to at least four of the most common reasons for stress on the job:

1. Poor communication, unclear or unreasonable job expectations and lack of resources within the organization.
2. Conditions which contribute to lessening of self-image (lack of recognition, feeling manipulated, etc.).
3. Ineffective personal attitudes (problems with authority, negativism, etc.) and poor peer relationships.
4. Lack of adequate knowledge and skills for work performance.

As the group gains in cohesiveness and makes use of the leadership potential of the group members, participants should feel freer to communicate their needs to supervisors and administrators.

The union of worker and supervisor as a cooperative problem-solving unit constitutes the second level of change. Many ideas will be generated in the ongoing communication within the staff group. In many cases the changes in attitude, increased motivation and innovative work procedures will enable group members to resolve some of the common problems mentioned above. However, there will be instances when the help of the supervisor is needed to resolve particular administrative issues. The role of the supervisor is to help supervisees accomplish work tasks and evaluate their performance. The educational and administrative elements of the supervisory role will be maintained in most organizations, as was true in the hospital setting. The union of supervisor and supervisee creates an additional force for the development of creative solutions to problems at work. In this situation, the supervisor and supervisee need to be open to the ideas and feelings of each other, recognizing that from each of their perspectives it is more possible to view the holistic nature of the problem. Too often it is a "one way street" — the supervisor talks and the supervisee listens. In a traditional administrative model, the supervisor is the person who has the authority and role responsibility to solve problems and make decisions based on his or her best judgment. In the proposed design, the supervisor will retain authority for decision-making but the supervisee will be involved in the process of problem-solving. In this way the interests of both administration and staff are served through their joint thinking.

The third step in the hierarchy of problem-solving involves key administrators who are able to conceptualize a situation from an even larger perspective. The thinking of this group should rely on the input of other staff who are attempting to solve a problem from within a particular range, such as an oncology floor or as an aspect of rehabilitation. The administrative group would consider the efforts of the second level — the supervisor and supervisee — and bring additional knowledge and skills into the problem-solving process. The composition of this administrative group would derive from the professional disciplines that were represented in the staff groups.

For instance, in the administrative group formed for the staff groups, members from nursing, rehabilitation, social work, personnel and training and education were represented, as well as the trainer for the project. The very fact that this administrative group was formed was a boost for the staff groups. It meant that persons in authority positions would listen to staff suggestions and it provided them with more impetus for struggling with the issues in their work lives.

PROGRESS OF GROUPS

Although the staff members were discouraged by not being able to resolve major problems, such as shortages of nurses on a floor, the groups did realize that they could help one another. Sharing of information about patients, giving and receiving support, identifying issues to discuss with supervisors and solving some procedural problems within their local areas were taking place. In some cases, members sought out other staff at the hospital to serve as a resource to help them address problems more constructively. The groups were judging their success on their ability to solve problems, perhaps because this had been an expectation in the training. Once they were able to recognize the equal importance of sharing feelings, supporting one another and building a caring social climate, the groups began to perceive gains from this part of their group experience as well as the task-centered aspects. They also focused more on areas of their environment that they could control and received satisfaction from these smaller accomplishments.

IMPLICATIONS FOR SOCIAL WORK
EDUCATION AND PRACTICE

Social workers and other caregivers in human service organizations will be faced with additional pressures to do more with less resources. Financial constraints will continue. The growing literature on burnout attests to emotional and financial costs to persons and organizations. The clients are the indirect causalities of staff ineffectiveness in dealing with stress. We are negligent about taking care of ourselves. The wellness programs that are being established for business and industry need to find their place in human service organizations as well. Perhaps social workers feel guilty if they take some time out for themselves. It is important to realize that staff are more helpful to clients if they are more fulfilled as persons and professionals.

It is suggested that we build in opportunities for social work students to experience supportive, problem-solving groups as part of their educational experiences. Some schools have similar types of groups that are related to work problems in the field setting (Walden & Brown, 1984). If we can instill the value of self and professional care during the years of education, it is much more likely that students who become professionals will continue the practice in their agencies. The resource of the staff person and the usefulness of the small group for creative problem-solving are valuable assets to develop wellness in the workplace. The client will obviously benefit from such a program to enrich staff. The social agency will also gain from these kinds of mutual help groups for its employees.

REFERENCES

Brown, L.N. (1984). Mutual Help Staff Groups to Manage Work Stress. *Social Work with Groups*, 7(2), pp. 55-66.

Cherniss, C. (1980). *Staff Burnout Job Stress in the Human Services.* Beverly Hills: Sage Publications, pp. 27-41.

Jackson, S.E. & Schuler, R.S. (1983). Preventing Employee Burnout. *Personnel*, 1983, 60 (2), pp. 58-68.

Lawler III, E.E. & Mohrman, S.A. (1983). Quality Circles After the Fad. *Harvard Business Review*, 63(1), pp. 65-71.

Naisbitt, J. Megatrends of '85: Reinventing the American corporation. *New York Times*, Section F, 23 December 1984.

Serrin, W. Giving Workers a Voice of Their Own. *New York Times Magazine*, 2 December 1984.

Tjosvold, D. (1984). Cooperation Theory and Organizations. *Human Relations*, 37(9), pp. 743-767.

Walden, T. & Brown, L.N. (1985). The Integration Seminar: A Vehicle for Joining Theory and Practice. *Journal of Social Work Education*, 21(1), pp. 13-19.

Yankelovich, D. & Immerwahr, J. (1983). The Emergence of Expressivism Will Revolutionize the Contract Between Workers and Employers. *Personnel Administrator*, 28(12), pp. 34-42.

Effects of New Integrated Methods Courses on Interest, Knowledge and Skill in Social Group Work: A Three-Year Study

Theodore Goldberg
Alice E. Lamont

SUMMARY. The paper reports the findings of a three-year study of the impact of curriculum change on interest, knowledge and skill in social work with groups. It compares students' experience in the previous method oriented curriculum with the present direct practice integrated curriculum. It also examines student interest in group work, their perception of group work skills and development of knowledge skill.

This paper reports the findings of a three-year study of the impact of curriculum change on interest, knowledge and skill in social work with groups. Social work methods content in the master's program at Wayne State University had been organized into tradi-

Theodore Goldberg and Alice E. Lamont are Associate Professors at the School of Social Work, Wayne State University, Detroit, Michigan.

tional sequences — casework, group work, community work — for many years. The sequences provided a "home" for faculty and students, a way of organizing students, advisors and agencies as well as a focus in selecting content for methods curricula. In 1982 the faculty voted to reorganize the curriculum at the MSW level into a first year "core" and a second year "concentration" plus "track" structure (consistent with Council on Social Work Education policy, 1982). The authors were aware of the debates about similar trends in schools of social work around the country and interested in the effects of such changes on the achievement of traditional group work objectives. Could measures of "gains" and/or "losses" be devised and assessed empirically? The authors seized the opportunity to study student responses to the curriculum before and after the changes were made over a three-year period: collecting data in 1983, the year prior to the change with the "old" sequence structure intact; 1984, the year of transition with a "new" first year core program and an "old" second year sequence curriculum; and in 1985, the first year of full implementation of the "new" core and concentration/track structure for all MSW students. Following discussion of the study design, major findings comparing group work in the "old" and "new" curricula are presented. The paper concludes with a discussion of the implications of these findings for social work educators and practitioners.

STUDY DESIGN

Data were gathered from students exposed to the "old" sequence structure in 1982-83 and from second year students only in 1983-84, the transition year. Their counterparts, students exposed to the "new" curriculum provided data during 1984-85 as well as while first year students in 1983-84.

Since first year classes are typically smaller than second year classes, (a result of the addition of BSW advanced standing students in the second year) all first year students were included in the samples during each of the phases. Second year students were selected with an eye toward balance and representativeness. Thus, all students specializing in Group Work, Organization/Community curricula and other smaller sub-groups were included together with forty to fifty percent of the casework majors. In 1984-85 the sample included all of the Macro majors and Interpersonal Track students were selected so that there would be adequate representation of the three Concentrations — a. Family, Children and Youth, b. Health and c. Mental Health. Responses were secured from 241 students (96%) exposed to the "old" curriculum and 242 students (92%) exposed to the "new" curriculum. In the remainder of the paper students who were exposed to the curriculum organized by sequences are referred to as "old" students and the sequence curriculum is referred to as the "old" curriculum. Students exposed to the integrated curriculum are referred to as "new" students and the integrated curriculum is referred to as the "new" curriculum.

The study is a longitudinal design with cross-sectional features. Three successive classes were surveyed as independent groups. Individual respondents were not followed over time. The design permits comparison of students exposed to old and new curricula. The very high percentage of participants results partly from the fact that the knowledge test was administered in classes and, while students had a choice, nearly all who were present participated. Student interest in the study resulted in high proportions (70% or better) completing the questionnaires as well. The samples are statistically equivalent to and very representative of student populations at the school during this period. In the old curriculum, better than 80% of the students specialized in the "micro" sequences of Social Casework and Social Group Work and a Generalist sequence offered in the second year.

The data were gathered through a five-page self-administered questionnaire placed in students' mailboxes which included sections on demographic characteristics, pre-school and school experiences and post-graduate interests. A brief test of familiarity with the group work literature[1] was administered in methods classes during 1982-83. It was supplemented by similar tests to assess familiarity with "micro" and "macro" literatures during the subsequent two phases. Apart from this addition, the same instruments were utilized throughout the study.

As noted above, one task was to devise means for assessing interest, knowledge and skill in aspects of social work practice. Interests were assessed directly by asking respondents to indicate which tasks they found most satisfying, which they hoped to practice on their first jobs and which they wanted to study following graduation. The assessment of knowledge and skill is more complex and approximations of these dimensions were utilized. Student skill levels were assessed by asking respondents to compare their skills in each practice category with that of their classmates rating themselves as "more," "less" or "as skilled" as most of their classmates. The authors believe that students know how well they perform in relation to others and are generally willing to share their judgements. Support for this belief is found in Radin's (1974) follow-up survey of Michigan graduates in which respondents' self-assessed skill levels were significantly correlated with ratings by their supervisors. The measure of knowledge utilized was the students' capacity to match authors with book titles drawn from group work, individual/family and organization/community literatures. Students were presented with a list of titles and a scrambled list of authors and directed to match them. The books/authors selected as "yardsticks" were those emphasized in the sequence curricula prior to the change. The authors of this paper do not claim that skill or knowledge have been measured. We believe, however, that these approximations are correlated with the dimensions of interest.

One further feature of the design merits mention. Questions related specifically to social work practice — types of prior work experiences, field work assignments, class and field faculty areas of competence, and future practice interests were specified in six tasks. Students were presented with the listing: Practice with 1. Individuals, 2. Families, 3. Treatment Groups, 4. Task Groups/ Committees, 5. Neighborhood Groups/Organizations, 6. Planning/ Coordination/Research (PCR) and could select one of these precoded items or a seventh "Other" category as a response. To illustrate, "In your *first* year field placement, in which of the above activities — was your field instructor most knowledgeable/experienced?"

FINDINGS

Pre-School Experiences

Since there was interest in whether student outcomes varied with exposures to differing curricula, it was important to ask first whether the two groups of students were comparable at the outset.

Thirteen variables were utilized in asking this question—age, sex, race, amount of prior social work/human service practice experience, amount of experience with the six tasks (e.g., individuals, families, etc.), whether they had been exposed to social work service/therapy, whether they were satisfied with that exposure and what modalities (individual, marital, family or group) were utilized. For all but two of these variables old and new students were equivalent. New students were more experienced in human services (62% vs. 48% had three or more years work experience; $X^2 = 4.88$, 1 df, p < .05) and there was a trend for them to have been more likely to be exposed to a variety of treatment modalities (31% vs. 21% were exposed to family, marital and group as opposed to individual services; $X^2 = 2.96$, 1 df, p < .10).[2]

While these differences are important to keep in mind, it seems clear that both old and new students are comparable in most respects. Of particular significance for this research is the fact that none of the sub-groups emerged as having had more experience in practice with primary groups prior to beginning the graduate program. Differences which might subsequently emerge are thus more likely to be attributable to the effects of schooling. The reader's attention is directed to the nature of these school experiences as reported by graduates.

School Experiences

Experiences in school were measured by asking students about their opportunities to practice the various modalities in field work, about the expertise of their classroom teachers and of their field instructors. The responses of students in the old and new programs are compared.

To examine opportunities to practice, the six practice tasks were listed and the students asked to indicate whether their opportunities to practice each of the modalities were: "None," "A Little," "Some" or "A Lot." For purposes of analysis the responses were dichotomized into high and low. Regarding instructors, students were asked to think of their classroom and field work courses and to indicate the areas in which their teachers were most knowledgeable/experienced using the six practice tasks as the structure for the answers.

In comparing the old and new students no significant differences were found between these two groups in either opportunities to practice with groups (e.g., 41% vs 35%, of the second year students indicated some or more opportunity to practice with treatment groups, p = NS) or perceptions of classroom teachers and field instructors' knowledge of this modality (e.g., 20% vs. 17%, perceived their field instructors as competent in this area, p = NS).

The effects of a specialized program in group work were evident in the three in-school experience variables measured in the old structure. Group Work majors were far more likely to report both opportunities to practice with treatment groups and teachers more familiar with that modality than other majors. However, when comparing all students in the old and new programs, there were no significant differences along these same three dimensions. It appears that in the area of practice with primary groups the competencies of personnel and opportunities to practice in field work courses remained about the same no matter which curriculum was in place. The impact of these school experiences on students in the two programs is examined in the next section.

Program Impact

Two questions are addressed in this section. First, what did the baseline findings indicate? How were the old sequence curricula working? In answering this question, Social Group Work students in the old curriculum are compared with classmates specializing in the other sequences. Second, what changes were found in the responses of students to the new curriculum? Were there evidences of program impact? In this case, all students exposed to the old sequence curricula are contrasted with students who began the program in Fall 1984 and were the first class exposed to the new Core and Advanced Concentration programs for both years of graduate study.

Beginning with the presentation of baseline findings, considerable evidence was found that the old sequence curricula were having intended effects — standards were in place (Goldberg & Lamont, 1983). Table 1 summarizes these findings. Students specializing in Group Work were more interested in that task, perceived their skill

TABLE 1

PROGRAM IMPACT: GROUP WORK VS. OTHER MAJORS IN THE "OLD" CURRICULUM

Variables	Group Work	Other Majors	Significance
Interests			
Very interested in practice w/treatment groups on first job.	46/52, 8%	40/110, 36%	$x^2 = 38.51$, 1 df $p < .001$
Interested in further study of group treatment following graduation	31/100, 31%	31/208, 15%	$x^2 = 16.23$, 1 df $p < .001$
Skills			
Perceived selves as more skilled in group treatment than classmates	27/53, 51%	12/107, 11%	$x^2 = 31.75$, 2 df $p < .001$
Knowledge			
High scorers on test of familiarity with the group work literature	39/71, 55%	10/156, 1%	$x^2 = 80.88$, 2 df $p < .001$

levels as greater and had higher knowledge test scores than did students specializing in the other sequences. Clearly, students who specialized in Group Work differed from their classmates in the anticipated directions. This is what would be expected given the greater opportunities to practice with groups, and exposure to teachers and field instructors more knowledgeable about group work. And, this is what was reported by Group Work students as part of their school experiences. These outcomes were not limited to Group Work majors. Respondents from each of the sequences in the old curriculum were, in general, more interested in, saw themselves as more skilled at and scored higher on tests of familiarity with literature in the area of their specialization.

The empirical examination of the old curriculum was viewed by the authors as the precondition for evaluating the new curriculum. What differences, if any, would be found? While one might expect programs to influence the knowledge, skills and interests of students, intentions do not always guarantee results. Having documented that Group Work (and other) Sequence program standards were in place, the central question of this project can now be addressed — is there evidence supporting fears about the loss to group work which results from the development of integrated methods curricula? Table 2 summarizes findings pertaining to this question. The outcomes do not point in one direction. To begin with, measures of *interest* in group treatment practice and in further study of that modality following graduation did *not* yield a longitudinal effect. Students in the new curriculum were slightly more likely to say that they were "very" interested in group treatment than students in the old curriculum although the difference was not statistically significant. So far as can be discerned from these data, interest did not diminish with the shift to a curriculum including methods courses in which group treatment is largely integrated with other content areas.

Perceptions of *skill* in this modality did differ when the two classes are compared, although the directions of the change are not visible in Table 2 which reports only on "more" skilled. Students exposed to the old curriculum were not as likely to rate themselves as "less" skilled (26% vs. 35%) and were more likely to rate themselves "as" skilled (50% vs. 38%) as their classmates. These dif-

TABLE 2

PROGRAM IMPACT: STUDENT RESPONSES TO GROUP WORK IN OLD AND NEW CURRICULA

Variables	Old	New	Significance
Interests			
Very interested in practice with treatment groups in first jobs.	86/162, 53%	108/187, 58%	X^2 = .78, 1 df p = N.S.
Interested in further study of group treatment following graduation.	62/308, 20%	84/347, 24%	X^2 = 1.59, 1 df p = N.S.
Skills			
Perceived selves as more skilled in group treatment.	39/160, 24%	50/187, 27%	X^2 = 5.70, 2 df p $<$ .10
Knowledge			
High scores on test of familiarity with the group work literature	49/227, 22%	9/197, 5%	X^2 = 15.82, 2 df p $<$ .001

ferences in responses of the two sets of students account for the trend towards statistical significance. In this area, the data point toward a slight drop in perceptions of skill in group treatment on the part of new students when contrasted with old. Of interest is the fact that this was the only practice task for which perceptions of skill levels showed evidence of change with the introduction of the new curriculum.

The clearest indication of change occurred in scores on the test of familiarity with the group work literature—the measure of knowledge used in this research. Scores were trichotomized (four to eight = high; two and three = medium; and zero and one = low) for purpose of this analysis; 22% of the old sequence students scored high in contrast with only 5% of the new students. Clearly, the students in the new curriculum were much less familiar with the group work literature.

For this School during the first years in which integrated methods courses were the rule, evidence was found that concern about the loss of group work has empirical support. New students were less familiar with the group work literature and tended to perceive themselves as less skilled with this modality. Interest, however, remained stable in spite of the curriculum change.

DISCUSSION

This research project had the purpose of testing empirically the consequences of what is now commonplace, but rarely tested, in social work education—the teaching of social work practice in integrated courses as opposed to the method sequences typical for the previous several decades. While data have been collected on each of the methods taught at Wayne State University, particular attention is paid in this report to the impact on group work—defined at this school as practice with *primary* groups.[3] In addition to the authors' long-standing interest in this modality, it is their belief that social work with groups could be more widely utilized by social work practitioners than is currently the case (Radin, 1974; Johns et al., 1978; Butler et al., 1982; Auch et al., 1982). (We believe the reason for the present state is that too few practitioners have competence and confidence in the use of the modality partly as a result of gaps in social work education. The expectations of many that integrated methods courses would lead to diminution of interest, knowledge and skill in group work drove this effort to measure what the outcomes really are.) In this concluding section of the paper, attention is paid to the meaning of the findings, their implications and some ideas about future research.

First, what do the findings mean? How does one make sense of what has been found? So far as can be determined differences in student "inputs" do not explain the study's major findings. Group Work students were much like their counterparts specializing in the other method sequences and old students were comparable to those exposed to the new curriculum. This is not the first effort to relate student background characteristics to their interests in various aspects of social work practice (Golden et al., 1972; Lauffer, 1971; Pins, 1963). These findings support the conclusion of other work in the area and suggest that social work students may be more alike than is sometimes thought when attempting to explain differences in program choices at the outset of training.

If students brought similar attributes and experiences, they were clearly exposed to differing programs in their schooling. Under the old sequence curricula Casework, Group Work, Generalist, Community and Administration students had different experiences. Of particular significance, in our view, is the clear demonstration of divergent field experiences corresponding to their sequence specializations. Also important is the finding noted in our first report (Goldberg & Lamont, 1983) and replicated in each phase of the study, that not *all* students appear to have the "right" experiences. While group work students have significantly more group treatment experience in their field placements than do other students, not *all* group work students had such exposure. For each of the sequence sub-groups, some majors did not have the chance to learn what the programs sought to foster. So, while standards were in place, there were students who seemed to "slip through the cracks" and the suspicion here is that this School is not alone in having such mismatches between school intentions and schooling programs (Dinerman, 1982; Hartman, 1983).

When the school experiences of students exposed to the new curriculum were compared with those who preceded them, differences were not as readily apparent as might have been expected. While it is known that some classroom courses were substantially revised in the new curriculum, the opportunity for students to practice with groups in the field remained essentially the same. Also unchanged were student ratings of class and field faculty areas of expertise with this modality. Since the "cast of characters" in both class and field were not substantially modified in terms of familiarity with group work when the new curriculum was introduced, these results are not surprising. Agency services don't change because schools alter their programs. Nor is it simple to make large-scale changes in the agencies utilized. Similarly, class and field faculty can, and probably should (Lewis, 1981), teach only what they know. Insofar as faculties remain the same, it is to be expected that students will perceive their competencies similarly.

An important question posed by the School findings flows from the overlap in the two curricula. If students in the new curriculum are exposed to similar opportunities to practice with primary groups in the field and perceive their class and field faculties as similarly qualified with this modality, as the findings indicate, what is the effect on group work with the loss of the sequence program structure? The opportunity to practice with groups in field courses and to be exposed to mentors with competence in use of the modality appears sufficient to sustain student interest. Overall, respondents to the new curriculum were just as interested in practicing group work in their first jobs and in further study of it as were students who completed the sequence programs. The loss of the sequence structure (and separate methods classes) did have an impact on 1. familiarity with the group work literature and 2. appeared to produce a trend for new students to see themselves as less skilled than their classmates. The reason for the drop in familiarity with the group work literature is apparent to those close to the new curriculum and its development. As the teaching faculty struggled to specify the "Core," the literature on group work was much less in evidence than had formerly been true. In part this seems a response to the absence of certainty about what to require (Dinerman, 1982) and the fact that faculty members with backgrounds in group work were, as is often the case, in the minority. They were simply outvoted when syllabi were being developed. Of interest, in this connection, is that when 1985 second year students were compared with second year students in 1984 who had taken the old curriculum, the new students showed statistically significant increases in familiarity with both Micro (X^2 = 8.26, 2 df, p < .05) and Macro (X^2 = 9.70, 2 df, p < .01) literatures. Thus the loss to group work was balanced by gains in other areas.

The outcomes of this study are: *group work interest and practice opportunities persist; familiarity with the group work literature and perceived skill decline.* We do not know if these findings apply in other programs or if they will remain true over time in this one. They do suggest areas for further work.

This project and its findings pose two questions at this stage of the analysis. First, to what extent is it possible to achieve the broader curricular objectives without the loss to group work documented above? It seems possible to introduce "corrections" to the new curriculum as these initial outcomes are documented and the School is gathering additional evaluative data at the present time. Course content and reading requirements can be modified. But important to underscore is that corrections guided by empirical data, of the sort presented here, are most likely to achieve the desired result. In the absence of such data, there will be limited agreement about what the outcomes of the new program really are.

The final question has to do with limits in the design and the data gathered thus far. Our interest was in finding out whether the quantity and quality of group work practice would be influenced by the shift in curriculum structure so common in social work education today. While quantity is relatively easily assessed, quality is another matter. How valid an indicator of knowledge relevant to practice are scores on the simple author-title matching task which was utilized? And to what extent are self-ratings of skill indicative of competence in practice? *Obviously, more carefully developed knowledge tests would be useful to all who aspire to assess the outcomes of educational programs in group work.* With respect to skill in practice, the authors are conducting a follow-up study of graduates exposed to the new curriculum. Will interest in group work practice persist following graduation? Does as large a percentage of the graduates exposed to the new curriculum practice group work following graduation as has been true of graduates in earlier follow-up studies (Johns et al., 1978; Auch et al., 1982; Butler et al., 1982)? Will the ratings of skill by supervisors of these graduates be correlated with self-ratings? These are some of the directions needing pursuit here and in programs across the country. In the absence of such data, we believe that all of us are "flying blind" when it comes to debates about what is a satisfactory curriculum for today's social work students.

NOTES

1. Copies are available from the authors.

2. Since a major question of this study had to do with the impact of change on group work a second set of analyses of the same variables was undertaken, this time contrasting Social Group Work students with students specializing in other method sequences in the old curriculum. In most respects no significant differences were identified.

3. The evolution of teaching of the method at W.S.U. resulted in an emphasis on primary/treatment groups in the Group Work Sequence. Practice with secondary groups has been given greater emphasis in the macro curriculum.

REFERENCES

Auch, Jean et al. (1982). *Further Explorations of the Job Market Experiences of 1978 and 1979 MSW Graduates*. Unpublished Master's Research Report (Detroit, Michigan: Wayne State University).

Buter, Jim et al. (1982). *Searching for Jobs: The Experiences of 1982 MSW Graduates*. Unpublished Master's Research Report (Detroit, Michigan: Wayne State University).

Council on Social Work Education (1982). "Curriculum Policy Statement for the Master's Degree and Baccalaureate Degree Programs in Social Work Education," New York.

Dinerman, Miriam (1982). "A Study of Baccalaureate and Master's Curricula in Social Work." *Journal of Education for Social Work*, 18(2), 84-92.

Goldberg, Ted & Lamont, Alice (1986). "Do Group Work Standards Work?" Paper presented at Symposium V, Detroit, Michigan October, 1983. Revised version to be published in *Social Work with Groups*.

Golden, Deborah, Pins, Arnulf M. & Jones, Wyatt (1972). *Students in Schools of Social Work*. New York: Council on Social Work Education.

Hartman, Ann (1983). "Concentrations, Specializations, and Curriculum Design in MSW and BSW Programs." *Journal of Education for Social Work*, 19(2), 16-25.

Johns, Carol et al. (1971). *Wayne State University Master of Social Work Gradu-*

ates: Follow-up Study of Work and Educational Experiences. Unpublished Master's Research Report (Detroit, Michigan: Wayne State University).

Lauffer, Armand (1971). "A New Breed of Social Actionist Comes to Social Work: The Community Organization Student." *Journal of Education for Social Work*, 7(1), 43-53.

Lewis, Harold (1981). "Are the Traditional Curriculum Areas Still Relevant?" *Journal of Education for Social Work* 17(1), 73-80.

Pins, Arnulf M. (1963). *Who Chooses Social Work When and Why.* New York: Council on Social Work Education.

Radin, Norma. (1971). "A Follow-up Study of Social Work Graduates with Implications for Social Work Education." Unpublished paper, University of Michigan.

Social Action Oriented Groups in Institutions for the Elderly: A Theoretical Framework

Carolyn Singer
Lillian Wells
Ranjy Basu
Leonarda Szewczyk
Alex Polgar

SUMMARY. This presentation will discuss a social group work model that integrates aspects of individual and group development, community development and social action for application with groups of residents, staff, and family members in institutions for the elderly.

This paper will discuss an integrated social group work model that incorporates individual and group development with aspects of community development and social action. The model was developed during a three year demonstration-research project for application with groups of residents, staff and family members in institutions for the elderly.

With institutions for the aged serving an increasingly older and more frail population the challenge is to produce an environment which enhances the social psychological and physical well-being of residents, with increasing efforts made to emphasize residents capabilities and potential.

Carolyn Singer, Lillian Wells, Ranjy Basu, Leonarda Szewczyk and Alex Polgar are members of the Faculty of the University of Toronto, School of Social Work, Toronto, Canada.

The goal of this project was to demonstrate a process of enhancing the social environment of institutions for the elderly. In the project we adapted the ecological approach of social work practice combining it with theory and strategies of community development and social group work to link networks of residents, their families and staff in institutions for the elderly.

The objective of this project was to involve the institution and its constituents in evaluating and improving the living and working environment. The project used a set of instruments developed by Moos (1979) for assessing the social environment of institutions for the elderly. Findings from this standardized assessment were then added to facilitate small groups of residents, staff and families to identify problem areas, set priorities, and develop solutions and strategies to improve the social environment in the institution.

The system had a long history of a hierarchical centralized model of administration. When the project began it was in the process of moving toward a more decentralized model with more autonomy and decision making possible in each home, but still with strong ties to central administration through consultants who were endeavoring to implement quality control while supporting initiative and creativity.

THE RESEARCH DESIGN AND INITIAL RESULTS

A pre-test, post-test comparison group design was used. Several homes were matched in the basis of the initial assessment and randomly assigned to demonstration or comparison status. There were two demonstration and two comparison facilities in the project.

The data analysis produced a profile for each home which described the physical and architectural features, policies and programs, staff characteristics and resident functioning and the social climate.

The initial results showed that generally minimal expectations were made of residents. Policies allowed for little resident choice or input. Greater emphasis was placed on residents' physical care than on their psychosocial state. Staff perceived residents as lacking the ability to be more active and autonomous. Residents were not encouraged to participate in planning for resident activity. Residents viewed themselves as not capable although they would have liked to express their feelings more openly.

These results indicated potential areas for change which were addressed in the demonstration phase.

THEORETICAL PERSPECTIVES

The following theoretical perspectives form the base for this model, which takes into account various concepts for social work practice.

Life-Cycle-Developmental Concepts

The project's perspective of the elderly residents is based on the concept of aging as a normal developmental phase in the life cycle, in a continuing process of growth and productivity, with certain life tasks to perform. In this concept of aging there is an emphasis on competence which allows for a continuing contribution to the environment.

Life Model Concepts

The developmental view of aging is congruent with Germain's (1979, 1984) life model, which provides the overriding conceptual base for this project. This approach directs its attention to people's transactions with their environment and works toward improving the individual-environment fit. There is a social action component in the life model with its change perspective, for individuals and for the social environment.

Generally the life model refers to direct social work practice on behalf of individuals and families. While using the life model as a base, this project has moved beyond the concept of advocacy on behalf of the client, and has engaged the client system itself in the advocacy process.

Social Group Work Concepts

Historically small groups were used as a means of enabling individuals to learn skills to increase self-esteem as well as improve their living environment.

Social work with groups is a model that addresses issues of individual development and control at the same time that group tasks are undertaken and implemented. Successful completion of tasks enhances both group and individual functions. The problem-solving model of social group work can operate creatively to generate many new ideas. People working together in a group can exert more influence that individuals on their own.

The social group work process incorporates the concept of participatory democracy. Grosser (1979) suggests that participation increases the individual's capacity to make contributions and gain a sense of belonging and control. The participatory process can be a device to keep human service bureaucracies aware of and responsive to client needs.

Community Development Concepts

Lewis (1983) sees social group work practice with adult community groups as a force in dealing with lacks in the social environment through increased citizen participation. There is the suggestion that consumers of social services have inherent power which can be activated to permeate bureaucratic systems, so that services may be more responsive as well as accountable to consumer needs. Lewis (1983) considers that social work had a major role in developing client skills to assume responsibility for taking action.

Organizational Change Concepts

Organizational change concepts suggest that a large system needs to institute problem solving structures in order to adapt to changes within the system and changes in the external environment. Implementation is facilitated through collaborative endeavors toward problem identification and problem solution which are supported and maintained by the institutional system (Brager & Holoway, 1978).

Social Action Concepts

Social action can be seen as a form of participatory democracy guided by knowledge, rationality and collaboration. Social action concepts also suggest that the achievements of social action groups can provide personal gains for participants (Glasser et al., 1974).

In summary, the above theoretical concepts have points of agreement and overlap. A synthesis emerged as the model for work with the groups in this project.

PREPARATORY PHASE

Prior to the formation of working groups to implement the project goal, each project social worker spent time in preparatory activities to become oriented to the home and to assess the home as an organization and as a community.

It was important to identify and connect with the power structure. A community development model was used in the reaching out process which introduced the project workers to the different sectors of each institution residents, staff, volunteers and families. Information about the project goals and the results of the initial data was shared with each of these population groups.

The project design called for the development of three committees in each demonstration home: a residents' committee, representative of different units and levels of care; a staff committee representative of management and line staff from the different departments and a joint resident/staff committee formed when residents and staff developed comfort and confidence in the project's approach.

The family committee was not part of the original design but was incorporated when family members expressed an interest in participating in the project. Family members represent a key social network for residents, and could speak on behalf of the mentally impaired residents unable to speak for themselves.

During this phase the project social workers noted those individuals who might be potential committee members and set criteria for selection of committee membership. Potential members were interviewed and members were selected on the criteria developed.

GROUP PHASES

Group development will be discussed in terms of process, content, and worker role. The analysis of the process will be based on Kolodny's (1973) model, and Greenfield and Rothman's (1984) analysis of termination and transformation.

Pre-Affiliation

During the individual interviews members agreed to the committees' purpose of addressing broad issues relating to improving the quality of life in the institutional settings. Unlike many change-oriented groups where the impetus stems from the group members who believe they are capable of taking action (Lewis, 1983), in this instance, the impetus came from the project. Committee members felt unsure of their position and needed to build confidence and proficiency in using the group process to meet identified goals.

Results of the initial data were used as a catalyst to engage the committees in considering broader issues. Areas of strength and areas of concern were documented.

Helping people to feel at ease was important to free expression and discussion. An egalitarian structure was set up where each member's opinions and ideas were valued and each had equal power in group decisions. The issue of trust arose in both resident and staff committees as they expressed concern about the possibility that an individual member's free expression of ideas in the committee could cause negative repercussions in the system. Only the resident committees allowed their meetings to be taped.

In the resident and staff committees the members had to live and work together outside of the groups, and initially this restricted free sharing of ideas and disagreements. Pre-existing relationships which were brought into committee meetings were sometimes an inhibiting factor.

In this system, staff and residents were unaccustomed to participating in a decision-making process, nor were they accustomed to facilitative leadership. All committee members had difficulty with the responsibility and autonomy entailed in the problem solving approach. To accommodate the committees' developmental needs the project social workers found it necessary to move to a more directive role while facilitating autonomy.

The social workers maintained high expectations for member functioning, showing respect for their capacities. Resources were identified within the group as well as in the larger system and members were encouraged to utilize available resources for information and clarification. The importance of representation was emphasized as well as ways of sharing information and gathering opinions from other residents and staff.

Power and Control

Issues of power and control were played out in member-member and member-worker interactions. The workers' authority to control and limit the committee was tested and their expertise was challenged. Members appeared to seek proof that the worker would protect them against their own hostile impulses. The social workers were able to support the groups in their efforts to deal with conflict, encouraging open expression of feelings and seeking some resolution while holding firm to the stated purposes of the group.

Questions of representation, responsibility and autonomy were recurring themes which needed resolution for the groups' effective functioning.

According to Lewis (1983) the process of problem identification in such committees is often stormy and frustrating. This is part of the realization that members will be responsible for much of the work, and that solutions are not quick or easy. The worker needs to hold the group to careful exploration of an issue and its implications before taking a course of action. If the worker is able to help the group define a concrete issue with which they can achieve success in a relatively short period, morale and confidence will be raised.

Certain concrete tasks were identified related to orientational aids, to information about current policies, procedures and staff and departmental functions. The need to clarify organizational functions was evident in all groups, and gave them a point of departure in their assessment of the home.

Intimacy

During the intimacy phase the need for continual clarification of purpose was evident. There was continued testing of the worker's expectations of the group, as well as a continuing struggle with issues of conflict and control.

However, the development of trust and comfort did emerge. Intensified interpersonal involvement grew as members expressed their feelings more freely, and were able to become mutually supportive.

The staff groups arrived at this stage later than the others. With time members did begin to share some of their difficulties related to fulfilling group tasks, and began to speak openly, which led to a better understanding of one another and of the problems of their different departments.

It was during this phase that the groups came to grips with their tasks and moved into the decision making and planning stage. While continuing to work on concrete tasks, some of the groups began to move to considering issues such as the need for privacy. The groups began to believe that they were capable of taking action on their own and others' behalf, and that their efforts were legitimate (Lewis, 1983).

Differentiation/Cohesion

During this phase members became more accepting of others' differences. In particular residents with considerable physical disabilities were accepted and their ideas valued. Differences of opinion were seen less as power issues and were used constructively toward achieving goals. The staff group did not achieve the same degree of openness as the resident and family groups.

All groups began to examine more complex issues, such as that of communication within the institution. In all groups, solutions were planned and specific actions taken. There were surveys completed by the resident group, resources outside of the group were used for information and planning, documentation was completed.

There was more sharing of information between groups and within the total system.

Task accomplishment promoted a sense of competence in group members. With success the groups became more ambitious in their plans and better able to function autonomously.

The staff groups identified the value of connecting with the resident groups since both were addressing similar concerns, and the staff began to recognize the validity of resident input. The staff groups suggested meeting with the resident's groups as common goals were addressed. Initially residents were somewhat hesitant to share their concerns and opinions with staff. It was in the joint sharing of responsibilities that staff and residents developed a greater degree of acceptance and respect for one another. Although all the groups were new to the institution, this group was the most unique because of the equal input and responsibility of residents and staff.

WORKER ROLE

In all groups the workers functioned in the role of enabler facilitating the problem-solving process, encouraging and helping people to express their concerns, organize their thoughts, plan collaboratively to implement their plan, evaluate both the outcome and the process, and nourish interpersonal relationships. The degree of support and direction depended on the nature of the group. The more autonomous the group, the more supportive and directive the worker's role (Lange, 1972). As the groups worked toward defined goals the workers' role shifted to a less directive one. The worker acted as a resource person, and also taught skills in communication, assertiveness, collaboration, negotiation, and evaluation.

The social workers required skills in working with the bureaucracy and the institutional community as well as with groups and individuals. Skills in dealing with conflict were essential.

The workers needed to be steeped in the goals and the theoretical underpinnings of the project in order to define and maintain their own roles.

IMPACT OF THE DEMONSTRATION MODEL

The work of these groups influenced the system in a number of ways, resulting in changes in individual attitudes, behaviors, relationships, and self-concept; changes in the community related to heightened awareness of quality of life issues; improved communication between various sectors; and changes in procedures and policies within the organization.

Both the tasks accomplished and the process itself had great impact. As part of the process of working together toward common goals, residents gained skills in presenting their ideas and staff gained skills in listening. Staff perceived residents as more competent and residents gained self-confidence. Both learned ways of working through conflict by negotiation rather than avoidance. As residents understood the rationale for certain procedures and policies they felt more security and control in their lives. All groups developed a greater understanding of the complexity of any change effort.

At a more concrete level the residents' group improved orientation aids, prepared a booklet for orienting new residents and their families, worked with the Residents' Council to set up a Welcoming Committee for new residents, and held a survey to determine residents' need for privacy.

Residents learned skills in assertiveness, communication and problem-solving. They developed confidence and skill in speaking out in other groups. They interacted more with other residents and developed closer relationships with one another. Toleration of differences increased. Residents found the task groups to be mentally stimulating. In fact nursing audits show that residents who were participants in the groups tended to have a decreased need for nursing care. Management began to view residents as more capable, a dietitian invited residents to participate in a menu planning committee. Residents also became more active participants in fire safety committees and advisory councils.

By their very structure the staff groups initiated more management/line staff interchange, and provided status for line staff. Staff, too, developed skills in identifying and sorting out issues and in presenting staff needs to administration.

The joint committee was an important vehicle for promoting staff/resident understanding. This committee worked on improving privacy for residents, improving communication, and examining decision-making processes.

The family groups had a special impact. This was the first time families had met together to assess the home's functioning and to provide recommendations for improvement. These groups provided a conduit for better communication and understanding between families and staff. The family groups instituted general meetings for family members at which families and staff could have an exchange.

TRANSFORMATION

We hypothesized that the institutions might want to continue some aspects of the project when the demonstration was completed. Greenfield and Rothman (1984) state that in practice, groups often continue beyond the termination phase into a new phase of group development which they call transformation. In moving to this phase, the worker deals with the "dual dynamics" of ending and continuity, so that while identifying and responding to the meanings and feelings that are a part of endings, the worker also explores with the group the feasibility of alternatives to dissolution, This concept provided a relevant base for planning the ending of the demonstration phase of our project.

The project groups needed ample time to assess their process, their accomplishments, and their disappointments. They were them in a position to make a choice between termination and transformation.

The social workers facilitated the groups' use of the problem-solving model in making these choices. They explored whether they wanted to continue; why they might continue; what supports they would have within the group; what resources they would require; provisions for renewal; and a definition of their purpose and goals.

As each group worked toward transformation the social workers moved into an advisor/consultant role, assisting the groups in testing out their new roles by having members take over group leadership.

The plans for transformation were discussed with management and administration in each home prior to implementation. As the project ended each one had accepted a structure to engage staff, residents and families in assessing changing needs and expectations.

CONCLUSION

This project demonstrated an innovative approach to working with groups of different constituencies in an institutional community, with a mandate to work towards improvement and change. We devised an integrated social work model which tested and adapted several theoretical concepts.

Clients' capacities to advocate on their own behalf were demonstrated and this approach was instrumental in increasing residents' competence in many areas of life.

It was possible to incorporate and operationalize all of our theoretical perspectives within the social group work model. The groups provided a structure to work on organizational change concepts since they employed procedures to assess the organization's functioning and recommend adaptation to changing needs. The concept of moving from termination to transformation provided for integration of some of the project's gains into the institutional system, allowing for a continued thrust toward assessment and change.

This model was viable in revitalizing all sectors of a long term care facility in working towards a better quality of life for everyone in the system. It can be adapted for use in other long term care facilities.

REFERENCES

Brager, George & Holoway, Stephen (1978). *Changing human service organizations: Policies and practices*. New York: Free Press.

Garland, James; Jones, Hubert & Kolodny, Ralph (1973). A model for stages of development in social work groups, in Saul Bernstein (Ed.). *Explorations in group work*, Boston: Milford House.

Germain, Carel B. (Ed.) (1979). *Social work practice: People and environments: An ecological perspective*. New York: Columbia Press.

Germain, Carel B. (1984). *Social work practice in health care: An ecological perspective*. New York: Free Press.

Glasser, Paul, Sarri, Rosemary & Venter, Robert (Eds.) (1974). *Individual change through small groups*. New York: Free Press.

Greenfield, Wilma L. & Rothman, Beulah (1984). Termination or transformation? Evolving beyond termination in groups. Sixth Annual symposium on the Advancement of Social Work with Groups, Chicago.

Grosser, Charles F. (1979). Participation and practice? in Germain, Carel, B. (Ed.). *Social work practice: People and environments, an ecological perspective*. New York: Columbia Press, 305-325.

Lang, Norma (1972). A broad range model of practice in the social work group. *Social Services Review*, 46, 1, 76-89.

Lewis, Elizabeth (1983). Social group work in community life: Group characteristics and worker role. *Social Work with Groups*, 6, 2, 3-18.

Moos, Roudolph H. (1979). *Multiphasic environmental assessment procedures (MEAP): Data collection and scoring forms*. Palo Alto, California: Social Ecology Veterans' Administration Medical Center and Stanford University.

Ethical Dilemmas in Social Work Practice with Groups

Dorothy A. Seebaldt

SUMMARY: This paper discusses the process by which the worker can aid a group in making a free, responsible decision. Consideration of the systems (internal and external) which impact on the individuals and group involved in an ethical dilemma, and the value conflicts which the worker brings to the issue is examined.

The purpose of this article is to focus on ethical dilemmas encountered in social work practice with groups. As practitioners are well aware, such dilemmas are many and varied, and often quite sensitive in nature. Here are two such examples from groupwork practice.

Example one: You are working with a group of mentally impaired children in a school setting. One of the group members is a 12-year-old boy, Joe, who lives at home with his mother and older brother. Joe frequently acts out aggressively. One of the methods you use with the group is play therapy. One day in a group session in which anatomical dolls are being used, Joe reveals the secret that he has been and is being abused by his older brother. After investigation by protective services, it becomes obvious that Joe needs to be placed in a residential care facility since his mother must work afternoons and does not acknowledge the problem. This leaves Joe home alone with the abusive brother for most of the afternoon and evening. In order for the courts to override the mother's right to

---

Dorothy A. Seebaldt is an assistant professor of Social Work at Marygrove College in Detroit, Michigan.

care for her child, you must testify as to what Joe revealed in the group.

Example two: Susan, a 23-year-old group member, announces to the group that she has just found out she is four months pregnant. She also tells the group of her intention to have an abortion as soon as possible, since she is certain that the father is not her husband. She obviously does not want her husband to know. She is seeking group support and understanding. However, several members of the group speak out strongly against abortion and try to talk her out of it. The following week, the group is filled with tension. Susan doesn't mention her feelings about either abortion or her pregnancy, yet those opposed to abortion obviously exclude her from meaningful participation.

The first step toward resolving these, or any other ethical dilemmas encountered in social group work, lies with the self, with each individual worker's knowledge and awareness of self. (This is always crucial, but tends to take on added weight in working with children, the handicapped, the frail elderly, and other highly vulnerable populations, since there are many times in such cases when the worker must assume the role of protective guardian.) Such self-knowledge involves clarification of one's own values and feelings regarding the issues at hand. We recognize our own values and feelings on two levels: first of all in general, on the abstract level, and secondly, in the concrete. Self-knowledge on the general or abstract level is frequently more common, and usually easier to ascertain. For example, "How do I feel about withholding data? About not telling the whole truth?" or "How do I feel about setting the law aside?, about overlooking its infringements?"[1] It is in answering such questions put to oneself and in the owning of the innate awareness of such answers that a worker develops and grows in self-awareness and knowledge on the first level, that of the abstract.

The next level of self-awareness, the concrete level, is the one most frequently overlooked or avoided by a worker. This involves the "nitty-gritty" particulars unique to each specific problem in each specific group. Here the worker must come to terms with questions such as: "How do I feel about this problem in relationship to this particular group? This particular group member? The other group members? This unique situation?"[2] The nucleus of true differentiated self-knowledge grows from struggling with questions such as these. It is usually when a worker grapples with issues and questions at this more specific level that a person touches into his/ her own internal ethical dilemmas in the concrete. It is here, in the specifics of persons, place, time and situation that abstract moral principles and positions become real, potent, and often enough, highly sensitive. These personal dilemmas, which are endemic to human nature, usually center around the issue of following an ethic based on *law* versus following an ethic based upon *compassion* and *love*.[3] (These two are not always in opposition, and need not be. However, their tension is frequently experienced, especially in concrete, specific cases.)

It is imperative that we as workers deal with our own personal dilemmas before we can effectively facilitate any group or group member in dealing with their dilemmas. First of all, and most importantly, it puts a worker in touch with his/her own value system.[4] Secondly, working through our own personal dilemmas is often a catalyst for enabling the group to work through its issues and problems. The worker's dilemmas are often a key to, and congruent with the group's and individual's dilemmas. As a result, a worker who is willing to look at and struggle with his/her own value dilemma has begun a process which will have direct impact upon the group and its processes.

This leads directly into an aspect of worker awareness which is probably more often overlooked than either of the value levels previously discussed. This awareness involves the owning, recognition and sensitivity to one's position of *power* as a worker to influence the group in a myriad of ways.[5] Four of these ways will be examined here. First, the vulnerability of the group to the worker's power; second, the vulnerability of each individual; third, the fluctuations in a worker's roles; and fourth, the elusive nature of free choice.

First of all, each client group, in its own way, is exceedingly vulnerable and highly responsive to the worker. Often a group, will speak and perform in whatever way they think the worker wants them to behave. The group leader is the *authority* figure, and the group will often set up norms to please the worker. The cost of adherence to such norms is frequently high: the rejection or suppression of values, the loss of freedom, and the forfeiting of personal values, beliefs or integrity.

Secondly, each member of a group, as an individual, is highly vulnerable to the worker's authority, since each individual is simultaneously experiencing the influence of the group, the authority of the worker, and the group's sense of worker "clout." Hence, at any given time, in addition to the subtleties of internal personal pressures, a group member is also experiencing the complexities of group and worker pressures, thus severely jeopardizing individual freedom and true growth. As a worker, one must struggle to become increasingly aware of these pressures and of one's ability to align with, sabotage, enable, and in numerous other ways, influence the dynamics going on within the group.[6]

Thirdly, as workers we need to struggle for clarity from moment to moment regarding who our focal client is in this particular instance: an individual member, a subgroup, or the group as a whole? What is our proper role in this particular situation, and what is the value of this role to this focal client? Are we the protector, the enabler, the teacher, the clown, the parent? We need to have clarity about this because as group workers know so well, the focal client and the worker's role are interdependent. Clowns create audiences; judges require juries; gatekeepers produce sheep. Wherever we decide to focus our energies and place our influence, every worker's ultimate responsibility is for both individual and group integrity and well-being. Finding this balance and maintaining such an equilibrium is an art requiring clarity of insight about both self and others.

Lastly, as Social Workers, we are often the only human beings who present to our clients a variety of options and perspectives for their consideration. This is extremely necessary and good. It is one of the hallmarks of our profession. We attempt to treat each person with dignity, freedom of choice, and true respect for their life situation regardless of age, sex, history or behavior. We not only present, but represent, a *holistic* approach that is found less and less in our highly specialized society.[7] (For example, judges have one orientation, doctors another, school principals another, lawyers another, etc.). By the very fact that our problem-solving approach is more open and client-focused, more options are usually generated. This increases a client's ability to choose and to respond freely.

Interestingly, this increase of personal freedom can simultaneously decrease freedom. In presenting the client with a wide range of realistic options, the worker becomes "the expert," "the guru." The decision-making power is quickly ceded by the client, given up once again to the "powerful other."[8] Unless we are sensitive to and in touch with our power as workers vis-à-vis our clients, the very monsters which we work to overcome — unfreedom and self-loss — we unwittingly create.[9]

In concluding this section on self-awareness and its tremendous importance in terms of ethical issues involved in group work, then, three questions come to mind for consideration which can be quite helpful in trying to sort through one's own thoughts regarding a specific situation. Ask yourself:

1. What is the correct thing to do in this instance?
2. What is the expeditious thing to do in this instance?
3. What is the good thing to do in this instance?

For example, if you are driving a child to the hospital, and the child starts bleeding profusely, and you come to a red light at a clear intersection, the *correct* thing obviously is to stop. What is the expeditious thing to do, and, above all, what is the good thing to do in this case?

The answer to the first question is always based upon law, which we need in order to uphold and safeguard the common good. The answer to the second question is usually based upon saving: the saving of time, of cost, and of the worker's own "self."[10] This too is legitimate, since our energies are always limited. Yet it is the more elusive answer to the third question which we are impelled to seek, both out of fidelity to our profession and its Code of Ethics and, above all, out of fidelity to our own human personhood. Seeking the *good* thing in a particular situation of moral ambiguity is painfully difficult yet humanly freeing. It always involves a judgment call (at times contradictory to the dictates of law and expediency) and then the taking of responsibility for one's actions, perfect or imperfect as they may be.[11]

Everything discussed to this point focuses upon the worker and the necessity of personal awareness, clarifications, and truth within the worker regarding both self and the group. Such an internal process of self-realization and awareness is a prerequisite to any success in resolving ethical dilemmas.[12] The process of personal self-awareness, with all of its facets and points, will happen at times quite quickly and with innate spontaneity; in other situations it may involve a deliberate choice to attend to each of the areas of self-awareness mentioned. Whichever is the case, such internal awareness of self as self, and of self in relationship to the group is essential for group processing of its dilemma.

The second area to be focused on is the worker's role in enabling the group to articulate its own operative values. Here we must become facilitators,[13] helping the group and each of individual members to become aware of intersecting sets of values: those of the group; those of each individual within the group. First and foremost, this means that we must strive to create an atmosphere of openness and acceptance wherein each person feels free to express him or herself, and to unmask his or her own beliefs. This can be a difficult climate to maintain, particularly when a value-laden issue is confronting the group.[14] There are two processes, however, which can be of help in doing this.

First of all, we as group workers need to help the group name the external influences impinging upon them as they attempt to deal with this moral ambiguity. Often we as workers will have to start this process by naming some of these pervading forces that impact upon all of us. These include such things as the cultural mores and traditions of this particular group of people, societal laws and expectations, each individual's social class, economic constraints, familial values and expected behaviors, as well as personal mores, traditions, and sense of what is "okay." People need to be allowed to own these things in themselves and to recognize them in others.[15] We all need to laugh and cry *about* them, not *at* them, in order to claim which of them are vital and life-giving to us in this particular situation.

In addition, each group must go through a process of self-awareness quite similar to that of the leader. This involves focusing upon the concretes of situation, issue, and person within the context of this particular group. What are the feelings, attitudes, and values of this group and of its members regarding this issue and the individuals whose lives it affects?[16] For example, "Do children suffer from growing up in a dirty and disheveled home?

In order to get to the heart of such matters, it is frequently necessary to help clients reflect upon their more underlying and foundational values out of which their answers to such specific value questions arise.[17] What is the meaning and importance of life, humanity, belonging, loss and death to each individual and to this group as a whole? For example, "Does the need to belong to someone or something take precedence over personal integrity or well-being?" "Is loss—in its multiple forms—a worse evil than death?" People need to be helped to name these beliefs aloud both for the sake of the group and for themselves. Articulation of values and beliefs is essential to conscious ownership of them.

A crucial step which follows this individual ownership of values is that the group as a unit must name its ethic explicitly.[18] What does this group believe about loyalty, confidentiality and group pressure? For example, is it acceptable to use group pressure in an attempt to bring about change in one member's behavior? Does loyalty to this group mean that we protect one another's vulnerabilities in all situations? Is group pressure so strong that personal beliefs and values are routinely suppressed in order to conform to the group norms?" Do the group mores resemble an ethic based upon law (what is right), upon conservation (what is expeditious), or one based upon human responsibility (what is good)? Getting a group and each of its members to articulate their beliefs about such an issue will take time and patience, but it is essential to the successful resolution of any group issue, especially volatile moral issues.

The group then needs to consider its mores vis-à-vis the values of each of its individual members. This is a critical moment in group process where conflict may need to be resolved, dignity must be upheld, and the art of give and take can be learned in an integrative, realistic way.[19]

Many people, adults as well as children, never come to this level of moral awareness. There are three distinct ways in which people can be morally blind. 1. They have no realization that they have their own *personal* moral code, nor have they ever articulated it to themselves or others. 2. They are oblivious of the fact that every system with which they interact has its own moral code which is continuously impacting each person's life and behavior choices. 3. Groups themselves (families, nations, clubs, etc.) are ignorant of and so fail to name clearly, their unique value system.[20] More often than not, no one has ever asked either individuals or the individuals as members of a group to claim their values and the behavioral implications of these values.[21] As a result of this moral oblivion, personal and public respect for one's moral code is lost. Yet *every* human person and human system does have a certain set of values unique to them, and our role when confronting a moral dilemma is to help our clients, even children, become aware of their unique value framework, and to allow us, along with the group, to know what their values are. It is only when values are known that they can be respected. Otherwise, we as workers, and the group as a human system, can get into attempts to change values in our clients, individually or collectively, that we are judging simply upon external behaviors.[22] And the irony is that it is only when a person's values are regarded with dignity and care that one is free to refine those values. It is at such moments of respect that rigid stances can give way to truth, and that divergent options can be looked at with freedom.[23]

This brings us, finally, to the third area for consideration, namely, the dynamics of group-decision-making. At this critical juncture, it is essential that everyone becomes clear about two major concepts: 1. the meaning of *morality*; and 2. the meaning of humanity, of true human personhood. Unfortunately in our society, many people associate morality either with following a set of laws, prescriptions, behavioral codes, or religious rules or with being merely expeditious, as has already been mentioned. While these are concrete expressions of morality, none of them *are* morality, nor moral actions *per se*. Rather, fundamental ethical theory states clearly that to be *moral* is to be *truly human*, and that to make ethical decisions is identical to making human decisions.[24]

However, the problem with such a fundamental ethic is that being truly human, being a full human person, is *not* a given at conception, nor even at birth. We are born into the human race, it is true, but becoming truly and fully human is a lifelong task that requires environmental development, choice, positive regard from both self and others, and responsible use of our freedom.[25] (And it is precisely because of this freedom that we — any one of us singly or all of us as a group — can choose to live as animals if we wish.) Becoming truly human is not only a lifelong process but also an ongoing choice.[26]

Consequently, it is very important in searching for *human* options that workers understand what humanity is all about, and that we talk with our client groups about what the choice to be human and to live humanly involves. It is important to help individuals and the group to move beyond the level of "Do's and Don'ts," "Right or Wrong," to a level where they are able to realize, personally, the most basic elements of such an orientation toward human life. Human morality is a choice to respect *myself* as a whole, integrated mind-body person, concurrent with a choice to respect the integrity of society, especially of the communities of which I am a part.[27] Being truly human, then, always involves self-respect and self-love, both in the present and for my future; at the same time it requires social responsibility, respect, and concern for others. We can never become truly whole nor fully ourselves in isolation; part of our very humanness includes a social dimension.

Because we are simultaneously individual and social by nature, we experience the tension I mentioned above between law (which safeguards societal wholeness and order), and respect for each person as an individual with unique needs and wants. Nowhere are these tensions felt more strongly than within a small group setting. In every human life, and in every human group, this tension is experienced at sometime or other, as we struggle to seek after personal integrity and social wholeness.[28] It is the breaking of either one of these needed "wholenesses," interior or exterior, which we often term "illness"; such brokenness may be physical, psychological or social in nature.[29]

The ethical decision, the moral option, then, is a choice which upholds or increases the wholeness of each human person, both individually and socially. Once an individual or a group achieves this level of awareness, respect and love for both self and others, they are ready to look honestly at each of the options before them with freedom and sincerity. It is at this point that we witness the beauty of the human spirit, with its freedom to grow, to change, and above all, to love.[30] The art of compromise is experienced first-hand as group members learn to give the respect they have received; the freedom to love is born of this respect.[31]

Does it happen all of a sudden, as a result of one major incident? Usually not, though it is possible. More often, however, people come to this point slowly, through small steps forward. For example, changing the group's meeting time or seating arrangements— seemingly minor issues—are points at which human worth can be upheld.[32] No issue is too small or insignificant. The same art can be learned in a multitude of ways.

The rest is relatively simple. As stated previously, the group and each of its members need to look at all of the options open to them in this situation. It is usually helpful to articulate the options aloud. Then it is important for all involved to name the concrete pros and the cons connected with each of the alternatives before them.[33] In choosing any option, one always gains some things, yet loses others. Oftentimes this is a painful moment. It may involve the choice between the better of two goods or the lesser of two evils.[34] People need encouragement to ask these fundamental questions and listen freely to their answers: "Which of these options—all with assets and liabilities—will be more life-giving to me as an individual, to us as a group, and to each of us as members of human communities and society? Or which will be least disruptive to my human integrity, and to the integrity of this group and of those around us?" The answer to these questions gives us the most ethical decision and provides true resolution of the dilemma before the group.

Needless to say, it is often at this point of decision-making that individuals or even the entire group will try to get the worker to make, or at least to sway, the decision. We all know how it is done—appealing to fairness, aligning with authority, pleading ignorance, acting incompetent, to name only a few.[35] The greatest service, the most humane gift, as well as the best leadership we can give at this point is to return the decision making to the group and its members. By doing this, we are respecting them as truly human, upholding self-determination, gifting each person anew with his/her own freedom and empowering them to become whole and alive.[36]

REFERENCES

1. Dietrich Bonhoeffer (1955). *Ethics* (New York: Macmillan Publ. Co.), pp. 367-69.

2. Rodney Napier & Matti Gershenfeld (1963). *Making Groups Work* (Boston: Houghton Mifflin Co.), pp. 246-47.

3. Vincent Ryan Ruggiero (1984). *The Moral Imperative*, 2nd. ed. (Palo Alto, CA: Mayfield Publ. Co., pp. 100-02.

4. Gabriel Marcel (1964). *Creative Fidelity* (New York: The Noonday Press), pp. 229-30.

5. Sue Henry (1981). *Group Skills in Social Work* (Itasca, IL: F.E. Peacock Publ.), p. 105; Lawrence Shulman (1984) *The Skills of Helping Individuals and Groups*, 2nd. ed. (Itasca, IL: F.E. Peacock Publ.), pp. 88-91.

6. Shulman, op. cit., p. 296; Albert Alissi, ed., *Perspectives on Social Group Work Practice* (New York: The Free Press, 1980), p. 274; Ronald Toseland and Robert Rivas, *An Introduction to Group Work Practice* (New York: Macmillan Publ. Co., 1984), pp. 176-77.

7. Alissi, op. cit., pp. 64-71; 295-301.

8. Shulman, op. cit., p. 299.

9. Frank Loewenberg and Ralph Dolgoff (1985). *Ethical Decisions for Social Work Practice*, 2nd ed. (Itasca, IL: F.E. Peacock Publ.), p. 25.

10. Ibid., pp. 108-09.

11. Ruggiero, op. cit., pp. 83-85; Paul Tillich (1967). *Morality and Beyond* (New York: Harper & Row), p. 60.

12. Marcel, op. cit., p. 251.

13. Paul Glasser, Rosemary Sarri, & Robert Vinter, Eds. (1974). *Individual Change Through Small Groups* (New York: The Free Press), pp. 16-17.

14. Saul Bernstein, Ed. (1973). *Explorations in Group Work: Essays in Theory and Practice* (Boston: Milford House, Inc.), p. 105; Napier and Gershenfeld, op. cit., pp. 25-26.

15. Ruggiero, op. cit., pp. 13-18; Shulman, op. cit., pp. 85-87.

16. Shulman, op. cit., pp. 227-30; 246-48.

17. Ibid., p. 266; Bonhoeffer, op. cit., pp. 370-71; Marcel, op. cit., p. 52.

18. Shulman, op. cit., pp. 307; 312-13.

19. Napier & Gershenfeld, op. cit., pp. 203-08; Bernstein, op. cit., p. 105; I.D. Yalom (1970). *(The Theory and Practice of Group Psychotherapy*, 2nd ed. (New York: Basic Books).

20. Napier and Gershenfeld (1985). *Groups: Theory and Experience* 3rd. ed. (Boston: Houghton Mifflin Co.), pp. 113-21; 131-40.

21. Tillich, op. cit., p. 69.

22. Bernstein, op. cit., p. 101; Shulman, op. cit., pp. 307-08; Loewenberg and Dolgoff, op. cit., pp 12-13; Gerald Corey, Marianne Corey & Patrick Callanan (1984). *Issues and Ethics in the Helping Professions*, 2nd ed. (Monterey, CA: Brooks/Cole Publ. Co.), p. 266.

23. Shulman, op. cit., pp. 85-86.

24. Tillich, op. cit., pp. 28-48; Marcel, op. cit., pp. 75-77; Aristotle (1906). Nichomaechean Ethics, J. Burnet, ed. (London).

25. Erik Erikson (1950). *Childhood and Society* (New York: W.W. Norton); Lawrence Kohlberg (1976) "Moral Stages and Moralization: The Cognitive-Developmental Approach," in Thomas Lickona, Ed., *Moral Development and Behavior: Theory, Research and Social Issues* (New York: Holt, Rinehart and Winston), pp. 31-53.

26. Ross Snyder (1967). *On Becoming Human* (Nashville: Abingdon Press), pp. 50-73; Joseph Fletcher (1977) *Four Indicators of Humanhood: The Enquiry Matures* (New York: Hastings Center Reports 4(6), December), pp. 4-7; Carl Rogers (1961) *On Becoming a Person* (Boston: Houghton Mifflin); Marcel, op. cit.

27. Dietrich Bonhoeffer (1963). *The Cost of Discipleship* (New York: Macmillan Co.), pp. 112-14; Ethics, op. cit., pp. 49-54.

28. Ruggiero, op. cit., pp. 28-48.

29. Elfriede Schlesinger (1985). *Health Care Social Work Practice: Concepts and Strategies* (St. Louis: Times Mirror/Mosby), pp. 77-96.

30. Marcel, op. cit., pp. 104-19; 222-54.

31. Henry, op. cit., pp. 159-61; Napier & Gershenfeld, Groups, op. cit., p. 349-50.

32. Shulman, op. cit., pp. 187-188; Glasser et al., op. cit., pp 194-96.

33. Napier & Gershenfeld, *Groups*, op. cit., pp. 349-50; 462-463.

34. Ruggiero, op. cit., pp. 89-94; Bonhoeffer, *Ethics*, op. cit., pp. 214-17; 248-54.

35. Bernstein, op. cit., pp. 84-85.

36. Ibid., pp. 125-26; Marcel, op. cit., pp. 113-16. For the fullest source of documentation, see Dorothy Seebaldt, "The Development of Situation Ethics in the United States," Master's Thesis, St. Louis University, 1969.

ISSUES AND TRENDS IN GROUP WORK THEORY, PRACTICE AND EDUCATION

Breaking the Thought Barriers: New Frontiers in Social Work Groups

Gale Goldberg

SUMMARY. This paper focuses on developing an elasticized mentality, a mentality that can stretch far enough to see beyond the visible and think the previously unthought. For while the roots of social work with groups may be at Hull House, the frontiers are in our minds. Barriers to rubber-band thinking are explored; ways to get around, through, up and over them are discussed and areas of group work urgently requiring application of expansive modes of thought are identified.

It was a year ago that Judy Lee (1984) invited us to hear "The Message," by Grandmaster Flash and the Furious Five (1982)—the song that screamed from ghetto boxes across the nation, echoing the frustration and despair of those who played it over and over again, who lived it and live it still.

Gale Goldberg is a Professor at the Kent School of Social Work, University of Louisville, Louisville, Kentucky.

It's like a jungle sometimes; it makes me wonder
How I keep from going under
Don't push me 'cause I'm close to the edge!
I'm trying not to lose my head.

Listen.

Their warning that people will explode is very similar to the warning that Albert Einstein issued in 1946, less than a year after we dropped the nuclear bomb from the bomber, Enola Gay, and Hiroshima exploded. "The unleased power of the atom," Einstein told us, "has changed everything *save our modes of thinking* (italics mine), and thus we drift toward unparalleled catastrophe."

Today we are no further ahead in either the human or the nuclear domain. We have been warned about each, but we have not yet moved to avert disaster. Except for an occasional "No Nuke" sign, there seems to be collected denial of reality in the nuclear arms race. As a collectivity, we similarly deny the reality of increasing joblessness, hunger, homelessness, little to no available health care for those with low income and no income, the stress of hand-to-mouth living, loneliness, hopelessness, and so forth, pushing ever-increasing segments of the population to the breaking point. And when the people break, when the people finally explode from inside, *that* explosion will be more devastating than the blast of a nuclear bomb, for no one can stop the march of the dead. They have nothing left to lose.

To help them, the people pushed almost to the edge, and to help ourselves as well, *we must change our modes of thinking*. For if we do not, on the human front, as on the nuclear front, we will continue to drift toward catastrophe.

Our roots may be at Hull House, but the frontiers are in our minds. We can look back for inspiration and practice wisdom, but not for answers to the problems that confront us now. In fact, we cannot look for answers at all until we have posed the new questions—questions that are currently outside of our frames of reference and will remain so unless we do indeed step beyond our present cognitive schemes to "see" below the visible and think the previously unthought. Right now the problem is *how to think*, not what to do. That, therefore is the focus of this paper: vision and mind stretching, aimed at developing an elasticized mentality, a kind of expansive, rubber-band approach to thinking about social work practice with groups.

There is a story about Picasso that begins to illustrate some aspects of the issue. As the story goes, the husband of a woman whom the artist was painting appeared at the studio one day. Picasso showed him the almost finished portrait and asked, "What do you think?" Using all of the tact that he could muster, the husband said, "Well . . . it isn't really how she looks." "Oh? And how does she really look?" Picasso asked. The husband then took a photo out of his wallet, handed it to the artist, and said, "*This* is how she looks," whereupon the artist, examining the photo, replied, "Hmmm . . . small, isn't she!" (Hampden-Turner, 1981).

As the anecdote suggests, there are many ways to see and think about the world of people and events. We think differently when we work with groups, for example, than when we work with individuals. We actually "see" differently, formulate different perceptions from sensory experience, and differentially conceptualize what we see. When working with a group, our predominant search is for pattern. When working with an individual, on the other hand, our search is for the person, and our picture of the client at any given moment is usually taken with a zoom lens. When we work with a group, our attention is directed to the patterns of interaction among the persons, the properties of these patterns, and the locus and impact of each person within and in relation to them. Therefore our picture of the group at any given moment is and must be taken with a wide-angle base.

BARRIERS TO THINKING IN NEW MODES

Given this as a backdrop it seems reasonable to start dealing with expanding our modes of thought by examining some of the barriers involved, for beyond such learned and idiosyncratic differences in frames of reference as mentioned above, any attempt to think about thinking is fraught with problems. For one thing, language itself limits the concepts we can form. For example, we assign relationships among variables to one of four categories: cause and effect, correlation, coincidence or no relationship. Even in the face of overwhelming evidence of a relationship, such as seeing a license plate with the same digits as the address to which we are travelling and hearing that the same digits designated the winning lottery ticket that day as well as hearing the same digits in a phone message left on our answering machine that very day, our minds are completely boggled. And though it bothers us for a while, we finally, and probably improperly relegate it to the coincidence category. We do not have a word for such a phenomenon, and therefore we cannot conceive of it.

Beyond the limits of language, our knowledge, values, feelings and attitudes affect our perception, by creating expectations that further constrain us. That is to say, we only see what we expect to see. In Middleman's terms, "Believing is Seeing" (1983, p. 232) rather than the often quoted reverse of that. So, despite Hudson's statement that *successful* academic training is supposed to focus and restrict the meanings its students are free to perceive (1972), socialization into one and only one mode of thinking, the linear, cause and effect mode, places narrow parameters on the use of our intelligence.

There is also another way in which beliefs interfere with expansive thinking. If we believe a particular thing, then we do not probe further. Thus beliefs put an end to inquiry. A similar barrier to thinking in new modes is the one-right-answer approach ingrained in us by our early educational experiences, a process which led Neil Postman to quip, "Children enter school as question marks and leave as periods" (Postman & Weingartner, 1969, p. 60). And this attitude hangs on despite our intellectual recognition that life is ambiguous and that most of the time there are many right answers. There are two major ways in which this one-right-answer attitude stifles our impetus toward expansive thinking. First of all, if we assume there is only one right answer, we stop looking as soon as we find one; and secondly, having only one idea provides only one course of action, which can be fatal in today's world where survival demands flexibility.

If you have only one idea, you can't compare it to anything. You don't know its strengths and weaknesses . . . The French philosopher Emile Chartier hit the nail squarely on the head when he said, 'Nothing is more dangerous than an idea when it is the only one you have.' (von Oech, 1983, p. 24)

To bring this closer to home, perhaps twenty years ago people in social work education had the idea that it was possible to teach, in one course, something called "social work practice with individuals, families and groups." But, as we have begun to find out, the problem is that the instructor is often out of time before getting to groups!

Still another barrier to thinking the unthought is entrapment in Plato's logical paradox that says *without* preconceptions, we cannot recognize, therefore cannot seek the new. But *with* preconceptions we cannot find anything that is new. Clearly, this presents a cognitive bind. There are, however, some ways to think around, through, up and over some of these barriers, ways such as probing the beliefs with which we have become perhaps too comfortable, not settling for only one answer or one idea, supplementing words with visual imagery, using metaphors, opening ourselves to the new if and when pieces of it come unbidden, and admitting that tacit knowledge does exist, which is to say, recognizing that we know more than we can tell.

THINKING AROUND, THROUGH, UP AND OVER SOME BARRIERS

The idea of linear cause and effect . . . is inherent in the structure of a sentence, where a subject acts by way of a verb upon an object, but this may be a very inadequate rendering of what is happening especially of mutual influences. (Hampden-Turner, 1981, p. 8)

Despite the fact that mutual influence and mutual aid are core aims and processes in social work with groups, their nature is very hard to communicate fully because the linearity of our language cannot encompass the non-linear parts of concepts such as mutuality. Hampden-Turner suggests that we can correct, at least partially, for some of this linguistic bias by supplementing verbal statements with visual imagery, an idea that Ruth Middleman and I have discussed and elaborated elsewhere in terms of visual thinking (Middleman & Goldberg, 1985), and have applied to both the teaching and learning components of social work education under the rubric "Vision-Stretching" (Goldberg & Middleman, 1975; 1980).

Perhaps the most profound difficulty that one encounters, however, even when purposely intent upon thinking in new modes, is that "There are problems the very nature of which thought is not equipped to handle . . . some problems . . . can only be approached by *an intelligence not bound by thought*" (Kramer, 1974, p. 3). And this goes hand-in-hand with the Platonic paradox mentioned earlier. That is, you can only seek the known, for if you seek the unknown, where would you look and how would you know when you found it? It is reminiscent of a joke my father tells about a man looking for his lost cuff link under a street lamp despite the fact that he dropped it more than a block away. The punchline is that he chose to search where there was more light! The problem is that it is not a joke. The same theme can be found in the lore of various cultures, including an ancient Sufi folktale about the hero, Nasruden (1972). You could only know that you found the unknown if you recognized it, and if you recognize something, then obviously you already know it, so it is not unknown. This is troublesome and discouraging, for the inevitable conclusion is that one can seek only the old. From my point of view, however, whether or not it is seekable, the new *can come unbidden* if come is receptive to it.

Such receptivity requires looking and listening with a passionate mind, a quality of attention that is fundamental to knowing. To attend in this passionate way," . . . *there must be an openness, an innocence*, a putting away of the old ideas so that possibly the fresh can come in" (Kramer, 1974, p. 4). The least one can do is to leave a window open so that the breeze can bring in new scents and new sense, new insights, thus new sights. Even if a window is open though, there is no guarantee that the new will blow in. But one thing is guaranteed. If the window is *not* open, the breeze will not come in. New thoughts do not visit where they are not welcome.

In addition to leaving a window open, one can invite the new through play. We can turn concepts upside down and inside out. We can turn them on their sides and watch what happens. Perhaps a fruitful starting spot with words themselves, for as I indicated earlier, language limits our concepts. In this arena, Bateson (1980) can tickle the minds of social workers in general and social workers who work with groups in particular. He changes the parameters of the context within which characterological adjectives such as *dependence, aggressiveness,* and *pride* have heretofore and far too long been defined. His position is that all characterological adjectives should ". . . derive their definitions from patterns of interchange, i.e., from combinations of double description" (1980, p. 148). He suggests that we think of ". . . the two parties to the interaction as two eyes, each giving a monocular view of what goes on and, together, giving a binocular view in depth. This double view *is* the relationship" (1980, p. 147). He goes on to say that it is nonsense to discuss a word such as "dependency" or "pride" as something inside a person, and he calls for a re-definition that captures the interactive roots of these terms.

> If you want to talk about . . . 'pride,' you must talk about two persons or two groups and what happens between them. A is admired by B; B's admiration is conditional and may turn to contempt. An so on. You can then define a particular species of pride by reference to a particular pattern of interaction. (1980, p. 147)

To do otherwise "shifts attention from the interactional field to a factitious inner tendency, instinct, or what-not . . ." (1980, p. 147).

In order to do what Bateson has done, i.e., shift a definitional context, he had to challenge the interpersonal context in which these terms were previously defined, and he had to destroy the idea that they are internal, personal predilections. Similarly, in the physical sciences, Copernicus had to destroy the idea that the planet Earth is the center of the universe. And Darwin had to challenge the *Bible* in order to advance his *Origin of the Species and Descent of Man.* It is as Picasso said, "Every act of creation is first of all an act of destruction." One must break out of a pattern in order to come upon or invent a different one. And to do that demands learning from, but not standing in awe of history and the norms of the day.

In our own field, by 1955, seven earlier social work organizations or entities had to be destroyed so that one NASW could be formed. A more recent example began eight years ago when some teachers and practitioners became concerned that group work knowledge and skills seemed to be disappearing from the armementarium of social workers, so they organized us, as we began holding and attending yearly symposia on social work with groups — no matter where they were held, in this country and in Canada, we are still coming after seven years. A remarkable thing? How about the fact that we do not come to look merely backwards and reminisce; rather, we exchange a surprising number of innovative thoughts and experiences with a broader spectrum of groups than we have ever before considered within our purview! And now, with the help of Betty Lewis' Scholarship (1985), we seem ready to challenge and destroy the idea that the generic/generalist orientation to teaching social work is sufficient preparation for practice. Our message is clear. A generic/generalist approach is not epistemologically enough. More education for work with groups must be included in the curricula of schools of social work.

Another disquieting problem that impedes expansive, rubber-band elastic thinking is the fact that we often have to unlearn what we know in order to learn, discover or invent the new. To free ourselves to "see" developmental stages in an open-membership group, for example, we have to temporarily set aside what we know about developmental stages in closed-membership groups. If we do not, on the one hand, we may try to force-fit the new phenomena into a previously learned framework, or, on the other hand, we may completely deny that there are any identifiable phases in open-membership groups. The capacity to temporarily unlearn in order to pen oneself to new sights and insights is similar to Middleman's (1979) ideas about developing skill in looking with planned emptiness. Cultivating such an attitude is not only essential to discovery; it is also crucial to undoing stereotypes that often lurk just below our conscious awareness and blind us to differences that make a crucial difference in how we ought best to intervene for real help to happen.

Beyond leaving room for discovery and dispelling stereotypes, it should be noted that temporary unlearning can also precipitate and guide invention. Gutenberg, for example, had to forget that wine presses only squeeze grapes. In addition to unlearning, however, Gutenberg's creative leap from the wine press to the printing press involved another element. His invention was predicted on a metaphor, and metaphor is perhaps one of the most promising avenues to new thoughts and insights.

A metaphor can be thought of as a cognitive map.

> Metaphors . . . connect two different universes of meaning through some similarity the two share. In doing so, metaphors help us to understand one idea by means of another . . . The key to metaphorical thinking is similarity. In fact, this is how our thinking grows; we understand the unfamiliar by means of the similarities it has to what is familiar to us. (von Oech, 1983, p. 36)

So the wine press brought us the printing press, and later the pants press, and still later the garlic press — all built on the same principle. The design of the first iron bridge ever constructed is similar to its wooden predecessors in that pegs, albeit iron ones, were used to hold and reinforce it. And it is not mere coincidence that the first locomotives were called "iron horses"; nor that the first automobiles were called "horseless carriages." In our field, the concept of "contract" (Schwartz, 1971) is a good example of the use of a metaphor drawn from constitutional law to invent a tool that has significantly advanced the practice of social work. Similarly, the concept of "feedback," so critical to our work, is a metaphor adopted from engineering. In fact, we use metaphors all the time, almost without noticing them. We have triangles and triangulation, circles, fish-bowls, gatekeepers, brokers, advocates, brainstorming, and so on. For purposes of unlocking our minds in order to think in new modes, the value of metaphor cannot be overestimated. When we ponder old problems or when new problems arise, one of the things that we can do is to try making metaphors out of them. In doing so we may open up a host of brand new practice tools (oops, another metaphor) and possibilities.

An inherent danger in the use of metaphors, however, is the ease with which one can get caught up in them and begin to assume one-to-one correspondence which, contrary to our purposes, can lead to force fitting phenomena into spaces that are too tight for them, or are the wrong shape. Take, for example, the phrase "running a group" — as if it were a machine! Or the statement, "We're having group tonight" — as if it were the dinner entrée. To minimize this problem and maximize the potential of metaphors to help us invent new practice tools, we have to consciously resist falling in love with them so that we're free to recognize the point at which any particular metaphor is no longer useful and should not be pursued any further.

Beyond leaving a window open, creating metaphors for problems and inviting the new through play, to think in new modes we have to acknowledge the existence of *tacit knowing* and value it as legitimate practice knowledge, even if that means blaspheming the Holy Empirical. Tacit knowing, as we know, refers to knowledge of particulars that we cannot itemize, that we know but do not know how we know, that we know but cannot tell. It is the part of a practice act that we can sometimes model, but cannot directly teach because we have no words for it. With respect to the significance of tacit knowledge, ". . . an explicit integration cannot replace its tacit counterpart. The skill of a driver cannot be replaced by a thorough schooling in the theory of the motor car" (Pauline, 1967, p. 20), for example. Nor can the skill of a social worker with a group be replaced by intensive study of small group theory. Tacit thought, including hunches and intuitions, is indispensable to creativity and, according to philosopher-scientist, Polanyi, admitting that tacit thought and tacit knowing do exist is the only viable escape route from Plato's sticky contradiction. In Polanyi's words,

> . . . for two thousand years or more, humanity has progressed through the efforts of people solving difficult problems, while all the time it could be shown that to do this was either meaningless or impossible. For the *Meno* shows conclusively that if all knowledge is explicit, i.e., capable of being clearly stated, then we cannot know a problem or look for its solution. (1967, p. 22)

On the other hand,

> . . . if problems nevertheless exist, and discoveries can be made by solving them, we can know things, and important things, that we cannot tell. The kind of tacit knowledge that solves the paradox of the *Meno* consists in the intimation of something hidden, which we may yet discover . . . (which means admitting) . . . that we can have a tacit foreknowledge of yet undiscovered things. (1967, p. 22-23)

He goes on to say that it is tacit knowledge that constitutes,

> . . . the metaphysical grounds which underlie all our knowledge of the external world. The sight of a solid object indicates that it has both another side and a hidden interior, which we could explore; the sight of another person points at unlimited hidden workings of his mind and body. Perception has this inexhaustible profundity, because what we perceive is an aspect of reality, and aspects of reality are clues to boundless undisclosed, and perhaps yet unthinkable, experiences. (1967, p. 68)

SOME FOCI FOR EXPANSIVE THINKING

When the atom was split, physicists discovered that sub-atomic particles did not follow Newtonian Laws. This created a knowledge crisis that shook the very core of the discipline. Now there is a knowledge crisis in social work with groups, precipitated, in large measure, by diminishing resources. To stay out of the red, many agencies such as community mental health centers which are funded *per capita* have shifted to using groups as their primary mode of service delivery. Groups are a cheaper way to offer services since more insurance monies are collected per hour. And to keep the head count up, most of these groups have open membership. Although many substance abuse and chemical dependency programs have been using open-membership groups for some time, largely as a function of client reluctance to commit themselves to ten or fifteen consecutive sessions, open-membership groups did not demand our attention until their use became as widespread as it seems to be today. Schopler and Galinsky (1984; 1985), among others, have made a good beginning for us, but there is now an urgency to confront fully this knowledge gap that open groups present, for they do not seem to follow the same developmental phases that we identified in the traditional, closed-membership group. Probably open groups go through a cyclic rather than a lineal process, a process with recurrent returns to starting points coupled with continuous endings. Nevertheless, we still do not know how they develop, so the intervention models that were created for use in closed-membership groups may need to be expanded in order to guide practice in groups with open-membership. And this is where expansive thinking comes in. In order for us to develop the new theory and practice models necessary to understand the processes and guide intervention in open groups, and to do it well, we have to temporarily unlearn what we know about group development and intervention models. This is the way to "see" the new phenomena with open minds, to see them from a variety of perspectives, and invite new insights into their unique dynamics.

Another problem that arises and confounds traditional modes of thought about social work with groups is the fact that while groups proliferate, too often the worker with the group seems to focus on treatment of individuals while in the group instead of focusing on the group *qua* group. Increasing numbers of social workers are being called upon to do treatment with groups, in community mental health centers and elsewhere. The issue is that social workers in community mental health centers, despite the fact that they make up the bulk of the personnel, are following psychiatric models. This could be related to the fading of group work education from graduate social work program curricula, as well as reflecting the power structure of the mental health center.

If we do not teach the knowledge and skills that are essential to doing social work with groups, we are, in effect, sending social workers to seek direction elsewhere. Often they wind up doing whatever they watched psychiatrists or clinical psychologists do during stints as co-therapists in groups. Sometimes they devour and use the contents of inappropriate books that sport covers advertising techniques for making groups productive, most of which list one sensitivity-training exercise after another. And we cannot fault them for not doing what they were not taught to do in their schools of social work. Unfortunately, the ones who suffer are their unsuspecting and vulnerable clients.

In the hospital setting, group work is also on the rise. Here it aims mainly to help patients and/or their families to understand and cope with a variety of illnesses and disabilities. The groups are often educational and informational in nature and they are usually single-session affairs. These groups may not be done by the social workers at the hospital, however. The workers are often nurses who are increasingly interested in and educated to deal with counselling and groups. One can certainly wonder if social workers decline the opportunity these days because they have not been sufficiently taught how to work with groups.

It is no longer a matter of debate as to whether or not education for social work with groups should be revitalized in school curricula. It has to be done. More than likely, the issue is what will have to go in order to make room for it. And addressing this problem surely will require us to stretch our mental rubber bands. For example, NASW and CSWE are heading in a direction that emphasizes fields of practice. What if we discover this is the very content that could be eliminated and replaced by one, single course in how to learn a field of practice? In some way curricula must be adjusted, and any curricular change is bound to step on somebody's toes. But if the needs of clients take priority, schools have to turn out practitioners who are equipped to provide help through social work with groups. If not, *HELP* is in serious danger of becoming nothing but another four-letter, Anglo-Saxon word.

REFERENCES

Bateson, Gregory (1980). *Mind and nature*, New York: Bantam.

Goldberg, Gale & Middleman, Ruth R. (1975). Visual teaching: translating abstract concepts into visual teaching models. Paper presented at the Annual Program Meeting of the Council on Social Work Education.

Goldberg, Gale & Middleman, Ruth R. (1980). It might be a boa constrictor digesting an elephant: Vision-stretching in social work education, *Contemporary Social Work Education*, 3:3 (1980) 213-225.

Grandmaster Flash and the Furious Five (1982). Reprise Records.

Hampden-Turner, Charles (1981). *Maps of the mind*. New York: Collier.

Hudson, Liam (1972). *The cult of the fact.* New York: Harper & Row.

Kramer, Joel (1974). *The passionate mind.* Millbrae, Calif.: Celestial Arts.

Lee, Judith A.B. (1984). Social work with oppressed populations: Jane Addams won't you please come home? Paper presented at the 6th Annual Symposium, Advancement of Social Work with Groups, Chicago.

Lewis, Elizabeth (1985). Getting group work back in the curriculum and why. Paper presented at the 7th Annual Symposium, Advancement of Social Work with Groups, New Brunswick, New Jersey.

Middleman, Ruth R. (1979). Some particulars of urban social work practice and education, 1977. *The Urban Mission.* Louisville, Ky.: Kent School of Social Work, 29-39.

Middleman, Ruth R. (1983). Role of perception and cognition in change. In Rosenblatt, Aaron and Waldfogel, Diana (Eds.), *Handbook of clinical social work*, San Francisco: Jossey-Bass, 229-251.

Middleman, Ruth R. & Goldberg, Gale. (1985). It might be a priest or a lady with a tree on her hat or is it a bumblebee?: Teaching social workers to see. *Social Work with Groups*, 8:1, 3-15.

Polanyi, Michael (1967). *The tacit dimension.* Garden City, NY: Anchor.

Postman, Neil & Weingartner, Charles (1969). *Teaching as a subversive activity.* New York: Delta.

Schopler, Janice H. & Galinsky, Maeda J. (1984). Meeting practice needs: conceptualizing the open-ended group. *Social work with groups*, Summer, 3-21.

Schopler, Janice H. & Galinsky, Maeda J. (1985). The open-ended group. In Sundel, Marting, Glasser, Paul, Sarri, Rosemary and Vinter, Robert (Eds.), *Individual change through small groups*, (2nd Ed.). New York: The Free Press, 87-100.

Schwartz, William (1971). On the use of groups in social work practice. In Schwartz, William and Zalba, Serapio (Eds.), *The Practice of Group Work.* New York: Columbia University Press, 3-24.

Shah, Indries. (1972). *The exploits of the incomparable Mulla Nasrudin*, New York: E.P. Dutton.

von Oech, Roger (1983). *A whack on the side of the head.* New York: Warner Books.

Social Group Work:
A Central Component of Social Work
Education and Practice

Elizabeth Lewis

SUMMARY. This invitational paper charts the several approaches through which educators and practitioners have developed social group work practice. It reports on the current state of education for social group work practice, and outlines the rationale for greater emphasis and centrality for group work content in social work education. Finally it suggests several steps in achieving social group work method as an essential component in social work education and practice.

This paper argues for the increase of teaching social group work theory and practice in both undergraduate and graduate social work education. It identifies group practice as the pivotal arena in which the integration of personal and social foci (an historical dichotomy for the profession) can take place. It suggests a paradigm for practice within which the several discrete models or orientations may contribute selectively to personal and social functioning. It supports the argument by highlighting developments in the field of practice and in theory building for practice.

A brief history of the work of practitioner/theorist in identifying method is presented against the background of the developing social work profession. Evidence of the current state of education for group practice is provided. Finally, reasons for greatly increasing

Betty Lewis is Associate Professor, Department of Social Service, Cleveland State University, Cleveland, Ohio.

content on social group work in undergraduate and graduate social work education are identified.

The argument is based on several premises:

1. The method can be used to assist both personal functioning in primary groups, and the functioning of groups in the shaping and managing of the larger contexts of society.
2. The advancement of both theory and practice requires active involvement and cooperation between the academic and practice community.
3. The entity "group" is both the context for personal growth, development and change and the instrument by which persons can manage their social/societal responsibilities. Therefore, group methods ought to be central to education for social work practice.

STRUCTURE AND PROCESS IN DEVELOPMENT OF SOCIAL GROUP WORK METHOD

The current ambiguities in teaching social work practice with groups and the plethora of models, orientations and technologies, are confusing for the practitioners and educators, and these represent the current phase of an historic ongoing process.

In the history of developing the "profession" of helping people in their social relations, we have used a variety of organizing principles, derived from different intervention modalities and educational settings. The challenge continues to be how to create unity without diminishing the unique strength of diversity.

Early efforts at defining social group work practice included: 1. field of practice, 2. method, or 3. social movement as the central organizing principle. Currently (CSWE, 1983), group work method is subsumed under direct practice methods and is also identified as a field of practice. I am suggesting that social group work is a method, practiced in a number of fields and a basic ingredient in the development of social change. Integral to method is the worker's ability to focus on the integration of process and content, the how and why, the internal and external, the personal and social tasks and responsibilities. Exclusive attention to either dimension defines a different method.

SOME HISTORICAL DIALECT

The struggle for unity within diversity is evident in the membership of the early professional organizations, AAGW, that changed to AAGW. The NASWG, National Association for the Study of Group Work renamed in 1938 as AASGW, American Association for the Study of Group Work, changed its name in 1966 to American Association of Group Workers, or AAGW. It included practitioners in recreation, physical education, group work and informal education. Field of practice, agency and method all primarily focused on group rather than individuals. The settings framed the skills and purposes.

The similarities in settings provided an organizational base and enhanced efforts to study, define and improve practice with groups whose purposes were educational and social in nature and whose members needed opportunity to increase skill in the performance of social roles.

This effort paralleled the activities of case workers, psychiatric social workers, medical and school workers, community planners and researchers, each seeking to improve their particular and unique methods.

Although many schools of social work added content on practice with groups, some were either indifferent or hostile to the inclusion of this content.

The existence of the several "practitioner" organizations provided a vehicle for the advancement of practice, and perhaps a lobbying force with the schools of social work to include and update practice content. The merger into N.A.S.W. of all seven of these specialized professional organizations resulted in a shift from primary concern for the advancement of practice. N.A.S.W. expended its energy on the pressing concerns for a unified professional identity and more focused and effective efforts at influencing national social policy and legislation. A consequence of this shift, perhaps unintended, was the transfer of advocacy and action on public issues as imbedded in early group work practice, as the responsibility of worker with participants, to a professional organizational responsibility, carried by NASW through its newly created arm, PACE. As a result of this shift, group work lost its particular ability to negotiate and influence curriculum content on group practice within professional social work education.

Along with the loss of supporting structures at either the local or national level, the spread of practice with groups included a change in auspice. The focused treatment and rehabilitation agencies, in itself an indication of both versatility and centrality of the method, resulted in major methodological shifts. The integral mediating or interactive components of social group work practice in its wider context were relegated to peripheral attention. Social workers whose major method was case work found it more comfortable to use a group method which focused on working with individuals in the group rather than on the group as a whole.

Initial holistic conceptualizations of person-in-context, including the wider context of the group, the agency and the community; and the idea of the transferability of learning and skills from group to the wider arenas of life were diminished as the focus shifted to the psychodynamics of intra-group relationships.

In response to the shift of practice to new arenas, requiring new technologies, and perhaps because of the loss of a central channel for sharing the developments of practice, practitioners-turned-educators individually began extensive efforts to formulate group work practice models that were more congruent with the purposes of treatment agencies. In addition, prevailing and emergent social science perspectives such as behavioral, existential, phenomenological and systems orientations were added to the more prevalent ego psychological perspectives. This was an extended period of differentiation.

The need for greater sharing and integration of the diverse perspectives of social work practice with groups was met by the establishment of the Committee for the Advancement of Social Work with Groups in 1978. The annual symposia and the journal *Social Work with Groups* have become the major, but not sole vehicles for renewing dialogue, for encouraging research, and for examining the content on teaching of social work practice with groups. A brief review of current teaching of social work practice with groups is included later in this paper.

TRENDS IN CURRENT SOCIAL WORK EDUCATION: THE OPPORTUNITY FOR SOCIAL GROUP WORK

Exciting and sometimes controversial developments are occurring within social work educational institutions as well as in practice. In the early 1970s C.S.W.E. began to recognize the importance of undergraduate preparation for social work practice. The accreditation process has helped to develop standards and to identify general parameters of practice. At the undergraduate level there is commitment to a broad-range model of practice implied in generalist education, supported by an underpinning of systems and interactionist concepts. The centrality of groups in this generalist practice should be self-support.

At the graduate level individual faculty members have developed life model, holistic and ecological perspectives. C.S.W.E.'s project to develop primary prevention in mental health also contributed to a broadening of practice perspectives. Emphasis on family work includes attention to family roles, family process, family decision making, cohesion, all terms or concepts familiar to social group work practitioners. Knowledge and use of interpersonal and intergroup dynamics is on the increase, although not necessarily through the influence of social group workers.

These compatible trends within the social work educational sphere are matched by conditions in the wider society. The existence of numerous self-help, mutual aid and advocacy groups speak both to the universal recognition of the power of the group to support both personal and social change, and to dissatisfaction with services rendered by traditional individually oriented methods. Distrust of and disaffection with large complex service delivery systems suggest that consumers and provider organizations need a broader mechanism for their relationships than the single worker. Support groups provide one such mechanism.

The expectation is that organizations such as the Committee for Advancement of Social Work Practice with Groups will both aid in the development of practice knowledge and skill and be influential in advancing the teaching of this practice. Practitioner/educators must continue to be involved in the efforts to integrate and synthesize diverse perspectives on social group work practice models to achieve a broader and more inclusive paradigm. In this effort we need to look beyond the traditional auspices for practice to include those in which a group approach is the natural and necessary medium for service and to examine the use of group skills within an organizational, clinical and community context. To advance both education and practice with groups we need to incorporate both personal and social performance within one paradigm. This is both a theory building and teaching task. The educational institution should exercise its mandate and competence to lead.

CURRENT STATUS OF EDUCATION
FOR SOCIAL GROUP WORK PRACTICE

At the suggestion of the Committee for the Advancement of Social Work Practice with Groups a study of the teaching of social group work in the United States and Canadian undergraduate programs was undertaken (Lewis, 1983). A brief summary of pertinent findings follows: small group theory, models of practice, teaching modalities, texts and teaching resources, value issues, worker roles and responsibilities, contexts for practice, and practicum characteristics.

A re-examination of selected data raises questions about the usual response, "We already/always teach social work practice with groups." This is a factual assertion for many programs. However, amount of time spent, cohesiveness of content and congruence of classroom teaching with field practice experience is minimal in most cases. Graduates can be said to have knowledge about use of groups (not necessarily framed in social work values and constructs) and minimal skills in group participation, but they have not achieved capacity for skillful exercise of group work method.

The following data is drawn from 40 graduate programs (40/85 = 45.5%) and 87 undergraduate programs (87/300 = 30%) in the United States and from 10 programs (14/22 = 50%) in Canada. Data at the graduate level were compared with that reported in the 1982 and 1983 Council on Social Work Education (CSWE) studies,

"Statistics of Social Work Education in the United States," and were confirmed. These reports did not compile undergraduate data on this subject.

COMPONENTS OF CONTENT
FOR SOCIAL GROUP WORK PRACTICE

1. *Small group theory*. Small group theory is required in 71 percent of graduate and 93 percent of undergraduate but included in all programs. It is a separate course in 29 percent of programs, but elective in many. A small percent (7 percent) include it in HBSE, 31 percent combine it with practice and 32 percent use some combination of the above. Undergraduate programs combine it with practice more frequently than do graduate programs. Some respondents did not distinguish small group theory from social work practice with groups.

Although data suggest that students would have a solid base of small group theory, both time available and location of content in curriculum suggest limitations. A review of texts used suggests a further deficit; the "old familiars"; Cartwright and Zander, Hare, Bogatta and Bales, Olmstead and Hare, are hardly mentioned. Resources from psychology, psychotherapy, encounter, sensitivity and counseling, and social work practice texts which combine small group theory and social work practice dominate: Yalom, *Theory and Practice of Group Psychotherapy*; Corey and Corey, *Groups: Process and Product*; Johnson and Johnson, *Joining Together* are examples of the former; Hartford, *Social Work with Groups*; Heap, *Group Process for Social Workers*; Northen, *Theories of Social Work With Groups*, are examples of the latter. A range of generalist texts such as Pincus and Minahan, *Social Work Practice: Model and Method*; Anderson and Carter, *Human Behavior in the Social Environment*; and Zastrow, *The Practice of Social Work* also appear. This is not an exhaustive list.

2. *Social work practice courses and the teaching of social group work practice*. Four major approaches are utilized in teaching practice: by method; by field; by social problem; as generic/specific (or some mix). Of graduate programs responding, 41 percent use methods and 43.5 percent use a mix, with some methods being elective;

CSWE data is almost identical (42 percent methods). Undergraduate programs favor a generalist approach (40.5 percent), although 25 percent offer methods options. Combining all approaches, about 55 percent of BSW students have at least some small exposure to group practice. CSWE data (1982) indicate that only 0.8 percent of all graduate students were enrolled in group service courses. In 1983, 1.8 percent or 175/21,490 of students were primarily enrolled in group services.

3. *Models of practice*. Half of the respondents teach a model of social work practice. Significant differences emerged between program groups: only 30 percent of graduate programs specified a model, while 59 percent of undergraduates did. Graduate programs specified "bio-psychosocial," "ego psychological," and "ecological" and "life model"; undergraduate programs identified "system," "problem solving" and "generalist," with a few identifying "ecological" and "interactional." Canadian programs identified "social development," "generalist" and "life model." All these practice modalities may be congruent with group practice, but the amount of time given to particulars of group practice is difficult to estimate. The problems are intensified when practice is addressed in "micro" and "macro" packages, and faculty must teach individual, family and group practice within a limited time frame. It is thus difficult to assume any standard level of knowledge or skill in practice with groups among graduates.

An attempt was made to determine the extent to which programs taught a specific model of social work practice with groups, given the spread of orientations, emphases and borrowings from other disciplines. One third (33 percent) of graduate programs, fewer than 1 in 5 (18 percent) of undergraduate programs designated a clear model of practice; Gero's research (1982) identified four typologies, most having within-group therapeutic purposes, focused on individual change.

4. *Teaching modalities*. The axiom, "experience is the best teacher," undergirds teaching about groups. Both lecture and simulation were used by 75 percent of programs; over half used sensitivity training, especially in the undergraduate and Canadian programs, to sensitize students to their own participation and to the dynamics of selected group forces. It is not clear to what extent

worker role/interventive skill is identified in these experiences, or whether students can evaluate the appropriateness of these techniques in practice with groups. At times, students have confused teaching techniques with group work practice.

5. *Practice by content.* An attempt was made to cut across "models" or "methodologies" to identify any clustering with regard to practice concepts: a. group types, b. worker/group purposes, c. value issues, d. concern for context, and e. group developmental processes.

a. Of five group types, "client groups" were identified by 95 percent of respondents as most important and most frequently studied, particularly among graduate programs. Only 10 percent ranked other categories (self-help, task committees, adult community action and teaching-learning groups) as important to study.

b. Three categories of worker purposes were offered: 1. participation/client change, 2. group development, and 3. environmental change. Growth and development of participants was of most or major importance to 85.6 percent of the respondents; environmental change to 70 percent; and group development (especially group autonomy) to only 54 percent.

c. Of four values in social group work practice, the respondents indicated the degree to which each was explored: participation (64 percent), responsibility (55 percent), autonomy (40 percent) and equity (35 percent).

d. Exploration of linkage to contexts received relatively little attention. Agency purpose and sponsorship are explored by 93 percent of programs, but its significance is considered major by only half. Wider group linkages are important to only 10 percent, indicating that the increased interest in contexts evident in general social work literature has not been integrated into social group work practice teaching to any significant degree. This is a disappointment to those familiar with the roots of practice (Coyle, Wilson & Ryland, Phillips, Klein) and to those who would see group work practitioners and academics take greater leadership in advancing social group work professional knowledge and skill in dealing with the many contexts of life.

e. Of nine group development processes, all received high ranking. Overall group development is not an important worker purpose, but all respondents considered the internal dynamics of formation, contracting, decision making, conflict resolution, termination to be important. These processes are valuable to understand regardless of the ends toward which they may be directed.

Although the data may be classified as subjective and impressionistic, the areas provide a beginning profile of what is identified by teachers of practice as of importance in developing practice skill.

6. *Field education for social group work practice.* Students value the field practicum as their most significant learning, demanding their active "doing social work." Thus, the opportunity to work with groups should be of considerable importance to the development of practice skills. The study sought data on percent of students who had a field assignment with a group, approximate number of hours of direct work with a group, kinds of settings, and kinds of participants. Again, this data is approximate since respondents were not necessarily field coordinators.

The data suggest that many, if not most, students may graduate without any experience in group leadership, or with very minimal contact with groups. Over half of the students in 3 out of 5 programs receive no group work field experience. For these students with a field experience with groups, the actual time allotted varied extensively: 43 percent of the programs provided fewer than 12 hours; 21 percent, 14 to 40 hours; 19 percent, 41 to 75 hours; 17 percent, 76 to 99 hours. Graduate programs clustered at 10 and 90 + hours. Viewed against the overall requirements for practicum experience, students' exposure to groups may be as little as one observational period to as much as 10 hours per week of actual practice responsibility. Such competence as may be developed will be very idiosyncratic to a student within a program. Data from CSWE (1982) for graduate programs identified 321 students, or 1.5 percent who could be identified as in field practice group services. In 1983, figures are 255 (1.9 percent).

Since agency purpose/functions delineate the scope of practice, some exploration of settings for the practicum was undertaken. Overall, children's treatment institutions and community mental health agencies predominate. Graduate programs utilize community mental health settings, family agencies and adult treatment institutions. Undergraduate programs use a somewhat broader range: children's treatment, mental health, adult treatment, youth corrections, senior services, schools, family and neighborhood agencies. Canadian programs utilize health agencies as well.

THE STATE OF TEACHING

To summarize the state of social work education for practice with groups:

1. Social science theory about groups and group behavior is minimal and diffuse within the curriculum. There may be better "packaging" in multidisciplinary university settings which draw upon nonsocial work faculty to teach group theory. The time allotted within the HBSE sequence to small groups, neighborhood and community organizations and the wider contexts of society is overbalanced by emphasis on the bio-psycho-social focus on the person.

2. At the undergraduate level, the predominant "system" or "ecological" orientations expose students to interactive and multiple sets of relationships and social entities: the "generalist" model of practice provides the possibility (not necessarily the probability) of content on group practice. These are positives.

3. Content in group practice is concentrated primarily on within-group personal change objectives. Teaching modalities stress self-awareness, sensitivity techniques, sometimes confused with practice method. Dual leadership with an experienced worker is often the pattern for field teaching.

4. At the graduate level, patterns are diverse. The expectation that programs offer specializations produces field of practice/problem, or method/field combinations; individual approaches predominate. Group or community organization methods may be elective, or a major/minor selection may be offered.

5. Field education in practice with groups is totally inadequate. Time spent is too brief, parameters of practice as set by agency purpose are too narrow, field instructors are often not sufficiently skilled in social group work methods. Where agencies do use group methods, those who provide service are usually from other profes-

sions. The student has no clear practice model which is congruent with social group work practice. Field education in treatment, clinical and therapeutically oriented agencies predominate, and this tends to relegate group entity/larger context concerns to peripheral attention.

6. In both graduate and undergraduate education, time allotted to groups and to social group work is minimal. Many graduates continue to take courses, attend seminars, and enroll in institutes which are specific to their particular practice interests, even after two years of professional education. With minimal time allowed, the practitioner with groups will have developed little skill and even less confidence in his/her helping interventions. Finally, at all levels there appears to be little uniformity or agreement about what constitutes the core of social work practice with groups. There is no comprehensive paradigm. While there may be coherence within a given curriculum offering, there does not yet appear to be a common frame within either education or practice which encompasses the range of member needs and purposes, those of the sponsoring auspice, and encompassing professional expectations.

TOWARD A PARADIGM
WHICH IDENTIFIES CENTRALITY
OF GROUP WORK IN SOCIAL WORK EDUCATION

There are strong reasons for adding theory and practice with groups to all of social work education, even if one argues that clinical practice encompasses all of social work. If one includes prevention/education and support/experience in relating to and influencing wider contexts of life in an organized way as equally important goals to the daily tasks of the social work practitioner, we have additional reasons to increase the knowledge and skill in social group work practice.

Some propositions: 1. Overall, the social work profession claims as its field of expertise skill in aiding people to act purposefully, effectively and fairly with one another; 2. Human beings learn how to do this well or poorly, first, in the more intimate contexts or nets of relationships of family and kin and friendship and peer groups; 3. Depending upon how well people have learned to deal with issues of power and diversity, they are able to apply their skills to the tasks of mutual problem solving in the more complex public or civic arenas of life; 4. In order to maintain stability and at the same time provide direction to change, people must develop skill in assessing their current situation, identifying common interests, and developing a cooperative course of action that both satisfies them and does not infringe on the rights of others. They must be active contributors to society as well as recipients.

As O'Neill (1984) and the NASW Code clearly identify, we build upon two basic values: respect for persons and their dignity and worth, their capacity to govern themselves; and recognition of the need for a society which permits democratic participation and demonstrates caring for its members.

Beyond the family, the small group may be viewed as the first social context which offers the child a choice of belonging, participating. It offers the first experience of diversity of social attributes beyond those inherent in the family; of differences in power unrelated to parent-child and sibling relationships, although these too may be compared.

The small group is posited to be a major resource for monitoring changing circumstances and for generating new directions of social organizational renewal. The small group is at one and the same time context for interpersonal activity, learning and growth and instrument for expressing social perceptions and exercising social responsibilities. It deserves a position of central attention in social work education.

Specific Next Steps

Development of a broadened paradigm for group interventions is central to the task of persuading the educational community to increase and to center small group theory and social group work practice within undergraduate and graduate education. Such a paradigm will require exploration or societal processes of stability and change in greater depth, a greater understanding of dynamics of power, a shift in human behavior and social environment content to include more of small group theory.

We need to identify the field of practice within which group-in-context is the natural and primary focus for help. This will immediately open opportunities for employment and for influence in major arenas in life.

Community work, a major field of practice in Britain and Canada and basic to developing countries, is not identified in CSWE categories. Community work is, at its core, group work. It is practiced with tenant groups in housing estates, with low and middle-income residents in racially and economically changing neighborhoods, even with new condominium owners; with unemployed workers to help negotiate with complex corporations and the legal systems established to regulate the world of work; with vulnerable populations: the aged, handicapped, physically and psychologically abused, the displaced and impoverished.

A new professional discipline, urban studies, is emerging in higher education. Like community work programs offered without social work education, it develops knowledge about physical, economic and political processes but does not include methods of working with citizens to engage them effectively in decision making and dealing with group processes. An expanded social group work practice has much to contribute here. The focus of this practice with groups is aimed at assisting members and the group to develop such levels as they may sustain them in making mutually satisfactory working relationships with a range of formally organized systems, including the many complex organizations of the social welfare system: health, education, income maintenance, etc.

By identifying community work as a legitimate and fruitful field for social group work practice, we not only add numbers of heretofore neglected placement sites (often agencies and organizations which developed from the social movements of the '60s); we also open the profession to a student population which drifts to urban affairs, communications, law, public administration as alternatives to clinical social work practice. I think such a broad-range definition of social group work would be appealing to members of minority populations because it would fit more closely with their perceptions of life.

In reaching more broadly, we may yet achieve a more unified paradigm of social work practice with groups and find a receptive community of colleagues.

REFERENCES

Council on Social Work Education (1983). *Statistics on social work education in the United States: 1982*. Allen Rubin (Ed.), Council on Social Work Education, New York.

———(1984). *Statistics on social work education in the United States: 1983*. Council on Social Work Education, New York.

Hartford, Margaret E. (1962). Working papers toward a frame of reference for social group work practice. National Association of Social Workers, New York.

Lewis, Elizabeth (1983). The teaching of social group work: Update, exploration, comparison. Mimeo. Paper presented at Symposium V, Detroit, Michigan, October.

O'Neill, Maria Joan (1984). *The general method of social work practice*. Englewood Cliffs, N.J.

Wilson, Gertrude (1976). From practice to theory. Chapter 1, in Roberts, Robert and Northen, Helen. *Theories of social work with groups*. New York: Columbia University Press.

Toward the Quality
of Social Group Work Practice

Ruth R. Middleman
Gale Goldberg

SUMMARY. This article sketches a brief historical view of group work in social work and the move in social work education toward generic practice, away from a methods focus. Social group work and group therapy are compared and contrasted. Some standards are suggested for groups to qualify as social work practice with groups with special emphasis on the groupness aspect of groups. Some current issues such as open-ended groups, single session groups, co-leadership, self-help/mutual aid groups, and evaluation are discussed.

Practicing social work with groups today is like walking a tightrope. The task is precarious. Pressures of expediency, cost effectiveness, quality and thoroughness are hard, yet necessary to balance in these troubled times when people are hungry, homeless and unemployed; and when social programs receive assault after assault. More and more, it seems that the major appeal of groups in mental health centers and elsewhere, is that they increase the head count, therefore the funding.

In this review we shall sketch some key historical and theoretical developments in the view and use of groups. We shall differentiate between social group work and group therapy. We shall suggest a third form of social work with groups designed to help social group work adapt and survive in the face of current imperatives. Such an adaptation allows therapy and training to become the legitimate

Ruth R. Middleman and Gale Goldberg are Professors at the Kent School of Social Work, University of Louisville, Louisville, Kentucky.

content of social work with groups, provided they meet certain minimum standards which we shall suggest.

AN HISTORICAL SKETCH

According to Papell (1983), group work was a movement before it was a method. This movement involved persons from diverse callings: settlement houses, boys' clubs, Jewish centers, Ys, scouting, camping, education, recreation, church ministry, youth work and business. There were organizations: The American Association of Group Workers (1946). There were national meetings with exchanges of scholarly papers, and a journal, *The Group*, which lasted until the AAGW became part of the NASW in 1955.

Early group work concerns centered around acculturation of immigrants and rural arrivals to the urban scene, social reform, problems of social isolation as a function of industrialization, character building, leisure-time interests and skills, and recreation. According to Hartford, "the earliest definition of the group work process carried the value orientation of a commitment to social change" (1983, p. 758). In fact, it is group work that has anchored and continues to anchor social work in its tradition of social reform and concern for oppressed people, since much of casework shifted its focus to intrapsychic functioning (Briar, 1971; Lee, 1984; Papell, 1983). As Wilson indicates, we were "painfully aware of the deprivation of the people . . . served," and "never lost sight of the fact that institutional change was a prerequisite to actual relief of suffering" (1976, p. 11).

Coincident with and partly as a function of the shift in setting for social group work practice—from leisure-time to problem-oriented agencies (Tropp, 1978)—the late 1950s and 1960s witnessed theoretical advances in the form of discrete practice models summarized by Papell and Rothman (1966). The *social goals* model which they elaborate draws upon the work of several early theorists, including Coyle (1948), Kaiser (1959) Phillips (1957), Wilson and Ryland (1949). This model aimed to influence groups toward democratic values, social conscience, and social action toward the "common good"; to encourage socialization, and to enhance individual growth, development and learning. The *remedial* model, formulated by Vinter (1959), was grounded in psychoanalytic concepts, ego psychology and social role theory, and used the group to alter and reinforce individual behavior change. The *reciprocal* model, conceptualized by Schwartz (1961), was based on social systems theory and field theory, and directed the worker to mediate the engagement between the individual and society as each reached toward the other for their mutual self-fulfillment. This model introduced the terms *contract* and *mutual aid* into the vocabulary of social group workers.

At the same time, monies poured in for the War on Poverty, generating new service opportunities and new agencies as well as shifts in programs and neighborhood contact persons. While this generated excitement, it also created turmoil in the service network, especially since certain "outmoded" agencies were circumvented.

SOCIAL WORK EDUCATION

By the later 1960s and early 1970s, the trend in social work education, was to find, elaborate and teach "the generic," the underlying patterns of regularity that presumably unified the discrete practices of social group work and social casework. This effort was intended to define more sharply social work's identity as one profession. The outcome of this effort was catastrophic for social group work, as the supposedly generic was and continues to be weighted toward the side of work with individuals and families. According to Hartford, "we are reducing the content about small groups by *default* as we increase theory about individuals, families, social systems and organization — and have left small group theory as an elective" (1978, p. 12).

Obviously, the drop in social group work content from school curricula concerned several social work educators. It was Tropp (1978) who asked "Whatever Happened to Group Work?" and partially answered his own question in a substantial paper focusing on the ten years between 1966 and 1976. Citing statistics of the Council on Social Work Education, he pointed to the apparent paradox that schools of social work were dropping their specializations in social group work at the very same time that there was an upsurge in nation-wide enthusiasm for group-oriented experiences, especially of the sensitivity and encounter types.

MODEL DEVELOPMENT

There used to be group work agencies with which group workers identified. Group work in those days seemed to be a field of practice. Later, as we have described, group work was conceptualized as a method. Now, it would seem, group work is out as a method, but in as a field again! The most recent CSWE statistics classified group services along with child welfare, health, mental health, rehabilitation, aging, and so forth. And out of 21,490 social work students, only 175 (1.8 percent) in only eight schools, major in group services (Rubin, 1984). How did this happen? As indicated earlier, paralleling the decline in education for social work with groups, there was a staggering increase of 52 percent in generic methods sequences (Tropp, 1978).

Nevertheless, group work theories continued to develop in the 1970s. Much of the *social goals* model was incorporated with an existential/humanistic/phenomenological twist into the *developmental* model advanced by Tropp (1977). The *remedial* model evolved into the *organizational/environmental* approach (Glasser & Garvin, 1977) representing a broadening of the former boundaries to include concepts other than those strictly concerned with individual change. The *reciprocal* model became the *mediating* model and finally the *interactional* model (Schwartz, 1977). This name change reflected a shift in emphasis from the philosophical base of the practice to emphasis on the worker role, and from emphasis on the worker role to emphasis on the nature of the group process.

We will now compare and contrast social group work, group therapy, and a third formulation which we call social work with groups. This third formulation is more inclusive and more adaptable to the demands of current social and economic realities, client populations, and practice settings. Social group work flourished when schools of social work organized curricula around method orientations (casework, group work and community organizations). Social work students specialized in one of these methods; practice faculty were similarly specialized. This traditional form of social group work has been practiced largely in settlement houses, Jewish centers, Ys, and following these, in family and children's agencies, correctional institutions, hospitals, public welfare, psychiatric clinics, and public schools. Wilson characterized these group work agencies as "organized around problems of people rather than people with problems," by which she meant "the people-centered agencies attempted to help particular people with whatever problems they happened to have, while the problem-centered agencies offered help to people with particular problems" (1976, p. 7). Today group practice has shifted largely to the problem-centered agencies which used to be considered "host settings."

The practitioner typically was known as the worker—not the leader, not the facilitator. The term, leader, was a legacy from boys' clubs and scouting, while the term, facilitator, was a later import from humanistic psychology. Also, the worker did not *run* the group. Rather, she saw herself as an *enabler* whose job it was to help the group develop its own leadership and decision-making structure as well as to influence the development of democratic norms. She started where the group was, and as the group developed over time, she gradually became less and less central. At times she was an advocate. She directed members' attention to broader social issues which affected their day-to-day lives, and helped them to take appropriate social action. Sometimes she took the role of broker and referred persons with special need to other community resources. As her practice demonstrated, she valued self-determination, group autonomy, mutual aid, and concern for the "common good." While this traditional social group work was often therapeutic for group members, it was not therapy.

There are many group therapies, as Lang (1979) has discussed in detail elsewhere. In general, the practitioner uses the interaction of participants primarily for diagnostic purposes and as a means for generating material for the therapist and the group to examine. Group development is usually ignored. The practitioner is the expert, and as such, retains the central position in the helping process. She provides insights into the underlying psychodynamics of each party to any particular here-and-now exchange.

Even in a group setting, individual goals are held by each participant and/or for each by the practitioner. The participants begin as strangers to each other and for the most part remain strangers although they learn more about themselves over time and hear the others also learning about themselves. In fact, therapists often caution participants against socializing with each other outside of the group (Mullen & Rosenbaum, 1978), as this would contaminate the therapy process.

One of the most interesting things about therapy is the prestige accorded the word. It has definite appeal. Perhaps some social workers prefer the title "Therapist" since it connects them with psychologists and psychiatrists, and disconnects them from the social welfare arena and the poor. Perhaps they are therapists because of the great amount of group work pursued by the mental health (read illness) centers which are usually directed by other professions. Perhaps, too, therapy makes a service more marketable. The word, therapy, implies a need as opposed to a luxury, and people are more likely to be willing to pay for it, especially since the Growth Movement removed some of the stigma from seeking personal help for many adults. Clearly, the marketability and "professional" status account for the burgeoning expressive therapies — music, dance, poetry — which used to be known among social group workers as program activities. Take an activity; attach the word therapy; and presto! You are in business.

Along with the War on Poverty, the Civil Rights Movement, and the search for alternative life styles and community in the 1960s, the Group Movement appeared, This was often thought of as "therapy for normals," or more accurately, Growth Groups. Between the years 1969 and 1974, an estimated 5 million persons in the United States participated in one or another form of Encounter Group (also known as human relations group, training group, T group, sensitivity group, personal growth group, marathons, sensory awareness, and so forth). While these growth groups were often therapeutic, they were not therapy. They did provide instant intimacy at a time when alienation was a prevalent feeling.

To qualify as social work practice with groups, the work of the practitioner must include attention to helping the group members gain a sense of each other and their groupness. That is, they need to answer the questions: Who is here with me? What can groups do? And what are the possibilities for this group? From the outset, group members interact; for dealing with these questions elicits contributions from all to their work together.

First of all, to qualify as *social* work with groups, worker attention must focus on helping members to become a system of mutual aid. This comes about through encouraging between-member communication. A second criterion for inclusion in social work with groups is that the worker must actively understand, value and respect the group process itself as the powerful change dynamic it is. The power of group process as a change dynamic is confirmed by the small group research of Asch (1951), Crutchfield (1955), Festinger (1954), Shaw et al. (1957), Sherif (1956), and Tedeschi (1972). Group process includes both group development over time and the interactional process of each meeting.

The third criterion for social work with groups is a basic attitudinal set. From the very first group meeting, the social worker thinks about working herself out of a job. That is to say, she enables the group to increase its autonomy so that it can continue as a self-help-mutual support group after she either withdraws completely or changes her role to that of consultant or sponsor. This does not hold for groups of children or severely limited adults. In these instances, the worker helps the group to become as autonomous as it possibly can. Schwartz captures the essence of this special attitude in all of its shockingly humbling clarity: "The worker is an incident in the lives of his clients" (1971, p. 13). The life processes into which the worker "enters and make his limited impact have been going on for a long time before he arrived and will continue for a long time after he is gone" (1971, p. 13).

The fourth criterion is that the worker must help the members to re-experience their groupness at the point of termination. This could happen in several ways—verbal and/or nonverbal, e.g., joint reminiscing, or a final event.

Social group work clearly meets these criteria and can well be called social work with groups. Given our definition of work with groups, therapy can be the content and can be included also, contingent upon the way in which the group as a whole and groupness are used—in accord with our four criteria. This means that some clinical work with groups will fall outside the realm of *social* work, especially if the focus of the practitioner is limited to the treatment of individuals in a social context. Just as the legitimate content of social work with groups can be therapy, the content can be skills training, understanding life themes, or managing life transitions — structured groups where the worker is the expert until her knowledge has been imparted to the group (Middleman, 1980) so that members can continue to meet on their own if they so choose. A life-theme group is one in which members prepare for facing a common problem in their future, e.g., retirement. A life transition group, on the other hand, is immersed in coping with the life transition while it is occurring, e.g., new retirees learning to structure their days.

These additions — therapy as content and the structured group as format for content — are not intended to draw a circle that takes in everything currently done with groups by social workers. Rather, they are suggested in order to meet clear and growing needs.

Although our main concern here is direct practice, i.e., with clients, it should be noted that the knowledge and skills learned from direct practice with groups helps in work with agency task groups, team and other professional meetings, supervisory groups, administrative meetings, teaching, and functioning in professional organizations. While we do not see these people as clients, comparable dynamics and skills apply to the work.

CURRENT ISSUES

Open ended groups. Open-ended groups are gaining attention in literature and practice. This type of groups has a "constant turnover in membership, low cohesion and experiences some storming each time it adds or loses membership" (Hartford, 1978, p. 10). According to Henry (1981, pp. 306-318), when groups are open, there are three areas of practice that must be attended to: "the process of the group's recycling through stages of group development, dealing with the coming and going of group members, and sustaining the thread of what is the essential (or core of the) group." Hartford says "The worker will have to remain fairly central and provide continuity" (1978, p. 10). Galinsky and Schopler's study (1984) of 116 open-ended groups found they had multiple purposes: support (92 percent), problem-solving (87 percent), education (80 percent), and treatment (65 percent). There is clearly both a need and an opportunity for research and theory development in this area.

Single session groups. Single session groups are also gaining attention in the literature. Such groups include a session at a conference, a consultation visit, a one-time committee meeting, an intake group, and information giving session, a single session in a hospital or in a waiting room. Schwartz conceptualized a four phase process in working with groups and proposed that each phase not only applied to the total group experience, but to each meeting as well. These phases are 1. tuning in, 2. beginning, 3. work, and 4. transitions and endings (1971).

Co-leadership. There is considerable interest in, as well as concern for, the prevalence of co-leadership both in practice and in education for practice (Kolodny, Levine, Middleman, Galinsky & Schopler, 1980). Especially popular in other professions, co-leading is an import into social work: its very name (co-*leader*) is alien to social work's conceptual development, in that *social* work with groups, as we have pointed out, is not "run by" the worker, nor "led by" her.

Co-leadership seems important in open-ended groups in general, and often in the health area in particular where it is essential for the social work to team up with a nurse or physician who is more knowledgeable about the specific disease of problem in a technical way, and the roles of the two leaders are apparently defined.

Self-help mutual aid groups. Self-help mutual aid groups are not "an issue"; the issue here is how do or should social workers connect with them? According to *The New York Times* (Jan. 1, 1980), these groups exceeded 500,000, with Alcoholics Anonymous alone having nearly a million members (Gartner & Reissman, 1984).

In the early days, the self-help movement seemed to pose a threat to the professional community. In fact, a major impetus for the creation of self-help groups was the inadequacy many consumers found in some professional help models. Some persons at risk needed to establish greater self-determination and control over their personal and group destinies, to reduce monopolistic social controls by the professionals (especially in the medical care system), and to enhance the use of their own community's natural care-giving resources. These resources might come from the family, the extended family, informal friendship and workplace networks, religious organizations, neighbors, and so forth.

It is apparent now that certain persons may be willing to accept help only through the self-help mode. Moreover, as resources shrink for health and welfare services, the need for extended means of connecting with disparate populations in need of some place to consider their situations becomes increasingly important. Various professionals have come to find congenial roles in relation to these groups. They may do the initiating, provide consultation, training, make referrals to and from groups, convene conferences, conduct research, provide resources and publicity, and act as sponsor, a role especially valuable in the format of Parents Anonymous.

In recent years, many self-help mutual aid groups have added advocacy and social change initiatives to their support function. That is, they also focus on changing community attitudes, with particular attention to negative stereotyping. A classic example of success in this area is the elimination, in DSM III, of homosexuality from the mental illness category. Similarly, the American Association for Retarded Children became the American Association for Retarded Citizens. Many of social work's social action goals of earlier times now have special interest groups in their own right. Instead of duplicating, social workers can provide linkages to these groups.

EVALUATION

Evaluative research on group work practice is as necessary as it is in all other forms of social work. Arguments to the contrary seem to grow out of confusion about what constitutes empiricism. Those who equate empirical research with quantification either say it is impossible to do, or demand that we do in practice only what is quantifiable. It seems to us that both postures are dangerous and reflect a fallacious notion that experience which cannot be quantified is not empirical. We believe that experience over time *is* empirical, whether or not it can now or ever be quantified. Reason and Rowan similarly caution against "a flight from understanding in depth, a flight from knowing human phenomena as wholes," for "that means that the person, group, community *as such* is never known" (1981, p. xvi). For many social workers and for all social workers practicing social work with groups in accord with the four minimum criteria we have suggested, it is difficult to specify the independent variables, the interventions, let alone standardize them so there is a uniform basis for comparison. And outcomes, or dependent variables, are often just as difficult to specify. Some rough indicators of cohesion over time, for example, might be increases in humorous remarks, use of "we," decreases in put-downs, and so forth. These and other such group-related phenomena are countable, though the worker may not know what she/he did or did not do to produce the count. Also, the worker may not have time to count occurrences and still do her/his work with the group.

LOOKING AHEAD

To look ahead demands a swift glance around to see what is happening today in group work circles. Nineteen hundred and seventy eight was a banner year. It marked the beginning of *Social Work with Groups*, the first journal devoted to group work practice since the demise of *The Group* 23 years earlier. The second remarkable event in that year was a grass roots movement on the part of kindred spirits interested in a revival of attention to group work practice. This eventuated in the formation of the Committee for the Advancement of Social Work with Groups which has had seven annual scholarly symposia to date.

In a content analysis of articles published in *Social Work with Groups* between its inception and 1984, we found three major foci. Out of 188 articles 65 (34.5 percent) focused on diverse populations, including racial, ethnic and common-problem groups, e.g., residents on the Bowery, frail elderly, and recovering female alcoholics; 58 (30.8 percent) dealt with group work theory; and 15 (7.9 percent) were devoted to education for social work with groups.

Our findings that primary emphasis in *Social Work with Groups* concerned populations with special problems again reflects the impact of the economy on health and welfare services in both the public and private sectors. This is where funds are currently directed.

Currently money, therefore social service emphasis is focused on *adults* with *problems*, especially those problems that bring them to mental health centers, hospitals, clinics, nursing homes and geriatric settings. There is little money, therefore little time for outreach, and also little money for services to people believed to be "normal." Perhaps the most forgotten group is children with normal developmental needs which, paradoxically, formed the bulk of early group work attention. As Kolodny and Garland indicate, "group work practice with children . . . has been both a creative pacesetter and a neglected stepchild of the profession" (1984). Despite the recent "Year of the Child," the market has shifted from emphasis on normal children and activities to adults with problems and talk.

So far as the children are concerned, it appears that TV is filling a gap in lives that group work used to do. And older children frequent the video arcades, or play home video games or work computers. All of these pursuits (not trivial!) are essentially solitary ones. It would appear, that in the future, adults will need social work with groups to help them build the now neglected interpersonal relationships. Isolation, aloneness, and alienation produced by fascination with elec-tech will have to be countered by opportunities for group experiences.

REFERENCES

Asch, S. (1951). Effects of group pressures upon the modification and distortion of judgements, in Guetzkow, H. (Ed.), *Groups, leadership and men*. Pittsburgh: Carnegie Press, 177-190.

Briar, S. (1971). Social casework and social group work: Historical and social science foundations, *Encyclopedia of Social Work*, 16(2), New York: NASW, 1237-1245.

Co-leadership in social work with groups, *Social Work with Groups*, Special Issue, 3(4), 1980.

Coyle, G. (1948). *Group work with American youth*. New York: Harper.

Crutchfield, R. (1955). Conformity and character, *American Psychologist*, 10, 191-198.

Festinger, L. (1954). A theory of social comparison processes, *Human Relations*, 7, 117-140.

Galinsky, M. & Schopler, J. (1984). Practitioners' views of assets and liabilities of open-ended groups, presented at the 6th Symposium for the Advancement of Social Work with Groups, Chicago.

Gartner, A. & Reissman, F. (1984). *The self-help revolution*. New York: Human Sciences Press.

Glasser, P. & Garvin, C. (1977). Social group work: The organizational and environmental approach, *Encyclopedia of Social Work*, 17(2), 1338-1350.

Hartford, M.E. (1978). Groups in the human services: Facts and fancies, *Social work with Groups*, 1(1), 7-13.

Henry, S. (1981). *Group skills in social work: A four-dimensional approach*. Itasca, Ill.: Peacock.

Kaiser, C. (1958). The social group work process, *Social Work* (April), 67-75.

Kolodny, R. & Garland, J. (1984). Guest editorial, *Social Work with Groups*: Special issue, *Group Work With Children and Youth*.

Lang, N. (1979). A comparative examination of therapeutic uses of groups in social work and in adjacent human service professions: Part II—the literature from 1969-1978, *Social Work with Groups*, 2(3), 197-220.

Lee, J. (1984). Social work oppressed populations: Jane Addams, won't you please come home? *Plenary Presentations*, 6th Symposium for the Advancement of Social Work with Groups, Chicago.

Middleman, R. (1980). The use of program: Review and update, *Social Work with Groups*, 3(3) 5-23.

Mullan, H. & Rosinbaum, M. (1978). *Group psychotherapy*, 2nd ed. New York: The Free Press.

Papell, C. (1983). Group work in the profession of social work: Identity in context, in Lang, N. and Marshall, C. (Eds.), *Patterns in the mosaic*. Toronto: Committee for the Advancement of Social Work with Groups, 2, 1193-1209.

Papell, C. & Rothman, B. (1966). Social work models: Possessions and heritage, *Journal of Education for Social Work*, 2(2), 66-77.

Phillips, H. U. (1957). *Essentials of social group work skill*. New York: Association Press.

Reasoc, P. & Rowan, J. (Eds.) (1981). *Human inquiry*. New York: John Wiley and Sons.

Rubin, A. (1984). *Statistics on social work education in the United States: 1983*. New York: Council on Social Work Education.

Schwartz, W. (1961). The social worker in the group, *The Social Welfare Forum*, New York: Columbia University Press.

Schwartz, W. (1971). Some notes on the use of groups, in Schwartz, W. and Zalba, S. *The practice of group work*. New York: Columbia University Press.

Schwartz, W. (1977). Social group work: The interactionist approach, 17th ed. *Encyclopedia of Social Work*, 1328-1338.

Shaw, M., Rothschild, G. & Stickland, J. (1957). Decision Processes in communication nets, *Journal of Abnormal and Social Psychology*, 54, 323-330.

Sherif, M. & Sherif, C. (1956). *An outline of social psychology*. (Rev. ed.). New York: Harper and Row.

Tedeschi, J. (Ed.) (1972). *The social influence processes*. Chicago: Aldine.

Tropp, E. (1977). Social group work: The developmental approach, *Encyclopedia of Social Work*, 17th ed. 1321-1327.

Tropp, E. (1978). Whatever happened to social group work? *Social Work with Groups*, 1(1), 85-94.

Wilson, G. (1976). From practice to theory: A personalized history, in Roberts, R. and Northen, H. (Eds.), *Theories of social work with groups*, New York: Columbia University Press.

Wilson, G. & Ryland, G. (1949). *Social group work practice*. Cambridge, Mass.: Houghton Mifflin.

Index